THE THIN BOOK

HYPNOTHERAPY TRANCE SCRIPTS
for
WEIGHT MANAGEMENT

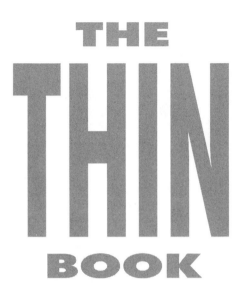

THE THIN BOOK

HYPNOTHERAPY TRANCE SCRIPTS
for
WEIGHT MANAGEMENT

HAL BRICKMAN, M.S.W.

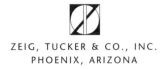

ZEIG, TUCKER & CO., INC.
PHOENIX, ARIZONA

Published by

ZEIG, TUCKER & CO., INC.
3618 North 24th Street
Phoenix, Arizona 85016

Manufactured in the United States of America

10 9 8 7 6 5 4 3 2 1

Acknowledgment

■

This book is dedicated to Dr. Daniel Araoz, whose supervision, support, and guidance have helped education transcend into inspiration. It could not have been written without having experienced the profound, unique and lasting influence of Dr. Araoz's ideas.

I am forever grateful to this great teacher and clinician.

Contents

■

Contents

Foreword

■

"Food, glorious food!" chanted Oliver with joy. And, yes, if food were merely a means to satisfy our hunger and to solidify our bonds with others, it always would be glorious. But food can also create problems, as it does in mostly affluent cultures: over-eating, undisciplined eating, eating for its own sake. The poor eat to live and often the rich live to eat. Hal Brickman, a psychotherapist with much experience, and even more sensitivity, common sense, and wisdom, approaches the problem of eating with a method that goes to the core of the problem: the mind's using negative self-hypnosis and convincing the person that consuming more food is good even when there is no physiological need for it.

Negative self-hypnosis explains many obsessive-compulsive problems, including addiction. After a while the person has developed a strong habit, "a second nature" by then, which, in itself, is difficult to break or change. But *underlying the habit* is the erroneous thinking that continues to justify eating in the face of satiety. This is what I called negative self-hypnosis, since it leads a person to repeat the harmful behavior with a sense of conviction. Brickman goes straight to that level: one's thinking. His test-proven scripts are all intended to transform the negative self-hypnosis into healthy self-hypnosis.

Several important principles, common in the New Hypnosis, dominate his work. First, patients are already experts in self-hypnosis, albeit negative. Second, hypnosis is a completely natural mental activity, without the need for artificial inductions or forced methodology. Finally, everything that happens in one's life (and in the therapy session, for that matter) can be used for one's benefit, as with the script for late-evening eating in Chapter 3.

Brickman takes a comprehensive approach, recognizing the metaphorical nature of the symptom. Many of the scripts address the unconscious meaning of irregulated eating. In this way, and by trusting one's unconscious, as Milton H. Erickson recommended, one's inner mind is invited to become aware of the reality, previously beyond the conscious control of the patient. In other words, Brickman uses many of these scripts not as magic cures, but as catalysts for serious psychodynamic work.

Still, today there is great ignorance about hypnosis, even among health professionals. The myths are not dead: the hypnotist takes control of the client's mind, the subject can be made to do immoral or hurtful things, only some people can be hypnotized, and so on. Unlike the traditional view of hypnosis, the New Hypnosis, which Hal Brickman uses here, involves the predominance of the imagination or right-brain activity, rather than logic and outward-reality orientation, or left-brain activity. On the other hand, for some traditionalists, hypnosis is the behavior that follows the induction selected and directed by the hypnotist, deemphasizing the role and input of the client, whereas the New Hypnosis, uses various diverse *spontaneous client behaviors* to facilitate hypnotic functioning. Those practicing the New Hypnosis do not believe that *they* hypnotize anybody. They simply guide the client so that he or she can use hypnosis for personal gain. When someone sees a hypnotherapist because he or she believes that his or her weight is a problem, the therapist helps the client to focus on the non-problem, the possible solutions to the problem. The solutions come from the client's own inner resources, which hypnosis is effective in tapping and utilizing, not from the therapist. Thus, in traditional hypnosis, the clinician is like a surgeon, whereas in the New Hypnosis, the hypnotherapist is a guide, a teacher, a facilitator, and a coach, as Hal Brickman demonstrates in his scripts.

The New Hypnosis approach is respectful of the client's individuality and personal life experiences. There are frequent invitations to consider associations and connections that come to mind while using hypnosis—memories and images from past events, people, places, and situations. This leads naturally to "the unconscious" and to aspects of the self of which the client was not aware, and that often explain the existence of such symptoms as irregulated eating, and, at the same time, mapping new roads to recovery. And because the client is considered an expert in using hypnosis, reframing and optimistic thinking are substituted for the negative elements of helplessness on which the patient has been relying on his or her own.

In talking about weight control, we cannot ignore the research findings popularized by Dr. Martin E. P. Seligman of the University of Pennsylvania, and president of the American Psychological Association. His oft-quoted "A waist is a terrible thing to mind" points to several eye-opening myths about overweight—the obese personality, the lack of will power, overeating itself, and the causal connection between the lack of physical activity and obesity—and zeroes in on *natural weight.* The fact is that each one of us, without knowing it, is bound genetically to stay within a specific weight range. Through hypnotherapy, the client is able to recognize the limits of natural weight and to accept it as part of the person he or she is.

Brickman offers hypnotherapeutic means to work effectively on the problem of weight management. Thus, *The Thin Book* is a welcome addition to the vast literature on this topic, and a significant contribution to the weight-management methodology and to the use of the hypnotherapeutic approach.

> Daniel L. Araoz, Ed. D., ABPP (Counseling Psychology and Family Psychology); ABPH (Clinical Hypnosis); Fellow APA; author of *The New Hypnosis;* Professor and Chair, Department of Counseling and Development, C.W. Post Campus, Long Island University.

Preface

■

Claire, a medical secretary, was frustrated and angry after three weight-management hypnotherapy sessions. She had come to see me to "get my waist back." She was about 30 pounds overweight.

Claire lived with her alcoholic parents. Her boyfriend, Larry, had recently "dumped her." She began our fourth session with, "I had a shitty week. I feel like a bad girl. I'm eating healthier foods since I started seeing you, but I still binge and devour food like it's going out of style." She looked at the floor. "I'm a goddamn eating machine."

Claire looked tired, and her eyes were sad. She said that she would start eating soon after arriving home from work. "It doesn't take long before I get restless and bored. Sometimes I have an empty feeling. That's when I miss Larry, and I feel so alone and despondent. And then the despondency turns into self-pity."

I asked Claire what usually happened next. She looked at her hand. Then she answered with a self-deprecatory laugh, "It's pig-out time and I'm the pig." Claire slammed her fist down on the arm of her chair. "Damn it! I cave in."

I asked Claire what it was that she caved in to. She looked up at the ceiling briefly and then at me, "I feel like I'm ruled by this infant in me who craves the nipple." "So you eat your feelings away?" She tightened her lips, slowly opened them, and spat out, "You got it."

After a short silence, Claire took a deep breath, nodded her head knowingly, and said in a quiet and certain voice, "I'm ready." She closed her eyes and welcomed hypnotic trance.

My sense of the clinical course to take was practically palpable. I reached for "Defense Against Feelings," a weight-management trance script that has been successful with many patients. It fit the context of this fourth session and of Claire's life. It was like reaching for a familiar poem that captures the essence of an experience.

The trance scripts in this book cover the most frequent challenges I have encountered as a clinical hypnotherapist specializing in weight management. Some clients, for example, eat too much too late at night, and others can't say "No" when someone pressures them into eating fatty food.

The scripts were carefully structured and sculpted, not only for speech fluidity, but also for metaphor resonance. The metaphors enhance the reprogramming of the part of the unconscious mind that is inhabited by the patient's saboteur. They use the teachings of the New Hypnosis, which believes that the patient's unconscious mind creates and fosters the poor eating habits by using "negative self-hypnosis," a term introduced by Dr. Daniel Araoz. Negative self-hypnosis is a spider's web of subterfuges and negative self-statements that reinforce harmful eating habits. The scripts use positive suggestions or positive hypnosis in the form of metaphors, analogies, empathy, and confrontation that contradict the effects of the unconscious mind. These interventions invite hope and educate the unconscious mind about adaptive ways to meet its core needs.

I find it useful, upon occasion, to give patients a copy of a weight-management script they can read at home. Here, the hypnotherapist functions as a distributor and as transitional object, a concrete reinforcement of the clinician's caring.

I suggest that you mold the trance scripts to the context of the session and the psychodynamics of your patient. Thus, you can embellish or delete whatever you wish to. It is best to read the trance scripts several times before using them. This will help you develop an increased presence, attitude, and delivery. The scripts offer a menu of options from which you can choose. This can relieve you of the pressure of having to come up with the most helpful trance for your patient.

Claire stretched and yawned. She rubbed her eyes and said, "I didn't want you to stop." "Why?" I asked. "I felt so peaceful and yet energized in a strange way. I saw a tiny yellow baseball. That was probably my unconscious mind. Then, suddenly it became a dark purple football that's handed to me in my gut. I hold onto it tightly. Then, I'm on this football field and I'm being chased by these very heavy football players I manage to outrun them to the end zone. Then I spike the football, feeling this sense of my own power."

I smiled, and let her unconscious mind digest the meaning of the imagery the trance script sparked and the time it needed to share what it had learned with the conscious mind. This leads to integration and the first hint that the process of growth is under way.

To Carol

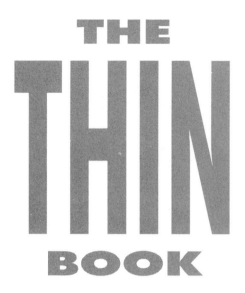

THE THIN BOOK

HYPNOTHERAPY TRANCE SCRIPTS
for
WEIGHT MANAGEMENT

1

■

Weight Loss for Those Who Have Never Been Hypnotized

Okay, _____, you don't have to think about hypnosis as such, but just about relaxing. And about focusing your mind so that you can use it more effectively. The name "hypnosis" is, in a sense, new compared with the fact that this type of mental-health practice has been used by people for centuries.

It's best to view it in a more natural way. And what is more natural than breathing? So focus on your breathing and allow your body to breathe . . . Find out which rhythm of breathing is the most effective for you, for your body right now . . . That's right, let your body find its own tempo of breathing . . . And while you breathe, let any tension be melted by the breathing. As if the breathing goes to that area that is a little bit tense right now. Softens it. And then melts it away. So breathing acts as a very soothing, natural way of allowing your body to function at its best.

And allow the breathing to bring your body to its highest level of effectiveness. You don't have to concern yourself with whether you are hypnotized or whether you are in trance or whether you are "under," as people say. Just enjoy what you're experiencing and, at the end, you're going to say to yourself, "Yeah, this is something different, a special way of using my mind, and this is called hypnosis."

There are many levels of hypnosis, as there are many levels of conversation, exercise, or any other activity. So with this in mind, and allowing your body to find its own rhythm of breathing, notice what happens . . . Your whole body seems to be slowing down. Calming down, because this is the natural outcome of gentle, rhythmic, natural breathing. And your breathing is the spirit of life. In many religions, the spirit is a name to define the mystery, the supernatural.

You want to be filled with that spirit of life. Of vitality. Of health and healing.

And with that, you can easily focus in on your body. And picture the body you want to have. Picture in very clear detail the body you know you can have. And maybe you imagine your body in action. Going up the stairs, or exercising. Maybe you imagine yourself at the beach, or in formal attire.

But you look at this new self and you are pleased with what

you see. And you know that that body can be yours. And you will become the creator of that new body. Starting with this clear vision in your mind of the body you want to have.

And you are focused on your goal, so that any distractions that may occur, you want to gently push aside. What you are doing at this moment is more important than distractions by noises or sounds or thoughts. And it's amazing how when we start relaxing, it seems as if some of the things that we have forgotten in the previous hours come to our mind. Things we did. Things we have to do. But you can gently push these thoughts aside and say, "I'll take care of that later. Now, I want to focus on this new self that I am going to create."

And it's almost as if you become the sculptor and the medium is your own flesh and blood. Some sculptors use wood or marble, but you are using your own body, your own flesh, to shape the way you want to be. The way that you know is good for you. The way you can be. And in order to accomplish this goal, you would like to think of the fact that your body is alive. Every part of your body, even now that you're resting and relaxed, is full of energy. Of movement. At the level of the cells, and even at the subcellular level, the atoms and the nuclei, there's tremendous energy. So recognizing that vitality, your conscious mind can become the protector of this wonderful, constant movement and change. And you may want to say to yourself, "I have only one body. I need my body to live, and to be in contact with the world. And I want to make my body last. I don't want to do anything that will interfere with the healthy functioning of my body.

"Consequently, I can develop a greater desire for the right type of food, and the desire for the wrong type of food can diminish. I want to keep my body in good functioning order and, therefore, I can exercise in moderation, according to my health. Also, I can exercise regularly, because that is beneficial to my body."

And visualize yourself selecting the right food . . . Visualize yourself enjoying greater satisfaction in the food that is good for your body. Imagine the colors and the shapes of that food. Imagine that food in your mouth; your taste buds picking up all the wonderful taste of the right type of food . . .

And just as you are breathing more naturally and more freely now, with your body feeling the comfort you are giving it, allow yourself to relax even more. An ever-deepening relaxation . . . And say to yourself, "This is happening now. My attitude is happening now, and once that thinner vision of myself is clearer, it's as if I have no other choice. Thinner is what I want to be and that's what I'm moving toward becoming."

And then, think of the real truth, that everything in your body is controlled by some area in your brain. So using your imagination, in a cartoonlike fashion, imagine that you are inspecting your brain. As if your brain were in a big laboratory. And inside that room, you will find the control center for hunger, appetite, and any inclination each person may have for various foods.

Are you getting the picture? And so, go to that area in this laboratory that **controls** the intake of food. Imagine yourself setting some sort of dial that will quickly warn you when you have consumed as much food as your body needs.

And next to that dial, you may find another dial that **controls** the taste and the enjoyment of food. So that you can set that dial correctly in order to **increase** the taste and the enjoyment of the right food, and **lower** or diminish the taste for the wrong food.

And since you have rearranged these ideas in your mind, visualize now how the effects travel to various parts of your body. To your mouth . . . To your taste buds . . . To your stomach . . . And to all the complicated areas of the digestive system . . . Very, very relaxed . . . Feeling that sense of well-being deepening even more.

And remind yourself that something is changing right now. Because the **body follows** the mind. And, depending on the thoughts we put into the mind, the body reacts. Depending on the thoughts the mind accepts, the body reacts.

And again, think of the body that you know you can have and the body you want to have. And the body you shall have . . . And you can say to yourself, "This is me. I have changed my mental image, my concept of myself. And, slowly, my body **becomes** what my vision **presents** to it. There is no other way. I will have the body I want. I will become what I want. I will be the artist. The sculptor who has created a new, wonderful, beautiful reality of myself, for myself. And with that, I want to promise myself that, yes, I want to practice this mind exercise every day. Consistently. Almost religiously. So that I can give myself a chance to **master** this approach, but also to experience its positive results.

"And I want to have this, 'yes', attitude. 'Yes' to health. 'Yes' to well-being. 'Yes' to energy. 'Yes' to good food. And the word 'yes' can remind me of my resolve, my expectation of success. So every time I think of the word 'yes,' or hear the word 'yes,' or read the word 'yes,' I can think, 'I expect success and I am going to **be** successful.'

"In order to make it easier for me to activate these thoughts. To **create** the body that I want, I can also use a sign, which would be a simple thing, such as touching my index finger on my left hand with my thumb. Just a secret that I have to remind myself of what I want to accomplish.

"And at times, I may be tempted to eat that extra portion of the wrong type of food, or even that extra portion of the right type of food, and my sign will refocus me on my determination. My resolve. On what I want to accomplish. On what I am accomplishing. Because I have started the process now and I want to continue it, until I see what I want to see. Because I expect success.

"And with this, I can bring myself back very gently, slowly, to the ordinary way of using my mind. Knowing that I now have the tools. The means to accomplish what I want. What I need for my body. My health. And, yes, my self-esteem."

2

■

The Resistent Part of Me

Okay, —————, allow yourself a few moments just to relax. Just to get in touch with your breathing . . . And to let that
breathing become very natural, very effortless . . . knowing that,
as time goes by, your body starts responding to the message from
your mind.

So with that sense of trusting your unconscious, trusting your
inner mind, where there is all the wisdom of survival. You want
to give yourself a few moments as a gift. As a present.

And the wisdom of your inner mind is what keeps you alive.
You don't know consciously how you are manufacturing, this

very moment, white blood cells and bone marrow. How you are keeping the optimal balance that keeps you healthy in your nervous system. In your bones. In your blood. But you are doing it.

And once you get in touch with this, you may experience a new sense of awe of or respect for your body. And, yes, your conscious mind wants to get rid of the extra weight. While your mind gains self-respect, satisfaction, and pride. But there is some other part of you that is interfering with that. That is saying, "No I'm going to eat more. I am not going to exercise." So instead of getting discouraged, you can recognize that we are not simple beings. Actually, when we say, "I do this," it's a short cut to explain too many complicated things. There is never "I." There is part of me. Part of you, the conscious part, wants to get rid of the extra weight. Have a healthier, stronger body. But there is another part that resists it, for whatever reason. And I don't know what that reason is. So you may want to imagine that part, because it's you also.

"And I want to resolve this ambivalence. This contradiction. Is it healthy for me not to get rid of the extra weight? Everything seems to say 'No.' So what is the fear that this other part inside of me has about losing the extra weight?

"And I can wait for the answer. Trusting my inner mind. What am I afraid of? What is stopping me from reaching that goal that in my conscious mind seems so attractive? What is stopping me from being the person I believe I can be? From having the body I believe I can have?

"No one is forcing me to eat more. Not to exercise. And I can give myself all sorts of excuses: lack of time, being in a hurry, not having the right food at hand. But I know better. So I want to just recognize that I have to own this other side of me. And by doing this, I'm going to make it much easier for myself.

"Because I can imagine myself as my conscious self talking to that other side of me that is perhaps stopping me because it is afraid. And helping that side to recognize that what my conscious mind wants is for the benefit for my whole self. Because my body is my responsibility and I want to take that responsibility seriously, but joyfully. So that I feel stronger. I live longer. I have more energy. All my organs are functioning healthier.

"And yes, there is a disagreement right now, but disagreements can be resolved. Especially, let's say, in a close family where there is love among the members. They can compromise and come to some sort of an arrangement. And that's why I say that this other part is not my enemy, because it's part of me. But probably is misguided. Is unclear as to what it wants. Is trying to be helpful in the wrong way. Like parents in the old days used to overfeed their children, thinking that was healthy. They meant well, but they were doing something wrong for the children's health.

"So the task for the next few days is to use this tape. Not just to listen to it, but to get **into** it. Also, to know that my conscious mind is at work all the time. So I don't know consciously the best time for me to have a complete understanding of this.

"I may be a little impatient and would like to have it right now. But I want to trust my inner mind and allow it to bring to my awareness what I need to know. Perhaps in my dreams. Perhaps during the day while driving. While doing something that doesn't require too much concentration. All of a sudden, a thought occurs to me and I say, 'Oh, now I know what it is!'

"But what I can do from a conscious point of view is to practice this mind exercise. Every day. And the change that I want is going to be a change for the better. So I can reassure my other part and say, 'Don't worry. It's going to be better.' Like the way a parent may have to reassure a child that moving to a new neighborhood is going to be okay.

"I'm moving into a new way of being. Which is going to be more constructive, healthier, happier, for my whole being. And with that in mind, I can relax a little deeper. I can go back to that image of myself. The way I know I want to be. And I can imagine myself already in the future . . . talking to that other part of me that used to be against this achievement. Recognizing how that other part agrees now with my conscious mind, and is glad that we have made the change. Knowing that the change is good for my whole being."

3

■

Late-Evening Eating

Okay, _____, take some nice, easy breaths and spend
a little time paying attention to the body and how the body re-
sponds to messages from the mind. After all, it is a double-edged
sword, in a sense. The mind can save us. And the mind can slay
us.

So at this point, the message from the mind is, "This is your
time. There is nothing else to do but . . . relax." And you can now
allow your normal relaxation response to take over, which is the
breathing. Gentle. Rhythmic. Easy. Smooth . . . Producing a

slowing down of all the systems in the body . . . And that's one of the aspects of relaxation.

And while you're becoming more in touch with your body, you may want to remind yourself that you, the adult conscious you, wants to take good care of your body. And distractions will come from thoughts, memories, things that have to be done later, or from external sources: sounds, changes of temperature, noises.

But you are now focusing your attention, narrowing your attention into this mysterious reality of your body. And it is mysterious, because it's so complex. There are so many things that are taking place every second of our existence in our bodies.

So you want to remind yourself, "I want to take good care of my body. But taking good care of my body at times becomes paradoxical, because what I want desperately may not be a good thing for my body. And I can think of a drug addict, who seems desperate to take (her/his) drug. And (her/his) adult conscious self knows that that is not good. Even though the body is yearning for it."

So you may have to remember that if you want to take good care of your body, at times you have to be a little tough with your body. Like a good parent has to be tough with a small child who insists on playing with sharp knives or scissors.

And so with that in mind, you may want to say to yourself that you want to start a new view of this issue. The sort of subliminal messages that food brings to our Being, "especially in terms of my experience. My experience has, perhaps by now, become like a habit. And as with all habits, it takes effort, perseverance, courage, repetition, to change the habit."

And I'm sure that you may allow yourself to think of some things in your life that you changed . . . habits of speech and in the use of grammar. Habits in driving, or manners, or ways of addressing people. And so many of the habits we have mastered, we have changed.

And so, this issue with food can be seen as a habit. "It can been seen as a habit that I want to change. On my way home, I may spend a little time thinking about how much I give during the day in my work. How many demands are made upon me. On my time. On my attention. On my knowledge.

"And perhaps, I want to spend a little time allowing myself to feel a little sorry for myself. And at that point, I can start planning how I'm going to make up for this. But in a way that takes care of my body. And I may find ways. I may promise myself a reward for the weekend. I may promise myself something that I enjoy doing, something I enjoy wearing.

"So I don't allow myself to arrive home without having thought consciously that, yes, the scales have to be even.

"I have given a great deal. I deserve something in return. But that something in return should be something that is good for my body. That is good for my health. That is good for my mind, my self-esteem. And again that's the paradox. Because I may have to accept the short-term pain for the long-term gain. And I can wait. I'm used to waiting for many good things in my life. So I can wait until the weekend.

"And again on the way home, I have to review briefly how I'm balancing work and play. Duty and enjoyment. If I start with that attitude, by the time I get home, I'll be more aware that the old habit will show its ugly head and I'll be desperate to eat. And not just to eat because my body needs it, but because I have to fill that hole in my soul, as it were. I've been drained. My spiritual blood has been sucked out of my being. And I feel that emptiness. But I know that I can replenish this in many other ways besides food.

"And that will be my challenge. How can I reestablish a balance through other means so that I don't use my mouth to fill myself when I feel empty? Instead, I use other resources that I have. And I want to trust my unconscious because my unconscious will give me some wonderful ideas.

"Some people go back to some activities that they have enjoyed in the past, but they have been too busy to enjoy now. Some people make it a point to do some physical activity, because it can be relaxing if it is rhythmic. Even though during the day there may be a lot of physical activity in the areas where I work, it's a tense activity, a rushed activity. Now I can go back to an activity that is rhythmic, soothing, quiet. But I want to remind myself that my unconscious can give me some good ideas. And what I have to do in my conscious mind is simply to remember that this old habit can be changed and that I want to change it.

"Even though it has happened in the past, I say to myself, 'This is the end of the line. I'm not going to let this habit take over my life at night.'

"And I want to visualize myself more aware. More ready. More prepared. More resolved. Because when I spend this time with myself, I am training for the real action. So the visualization is like a mental rehearsal. And I want to see myself, really, on my way home. Feeling bad for myself for a few moments. And then saying, 'I'm going to reward myself.' I'm planning something concrete. And that may make demands on me, because together with this habit, other bad habits very often have developed. (Like working during my free time. And many people in executive positions carry home work that they do during the weekend.)

"So part of changing this habit, in terms of the long-term gain, is checking any other habits that may be surrounding that central one, that of losing control of my food intake. And I want to imagine myself on my way home thinking gently about this. And saying to myself, 'I won't do this. I will do that.' And so on. I will relax. I will do some exercise. I will give myself a little snack that I have preplanned, something that is satisfying to me and healthy and good.

"And I can put that planning in slow motion. So that it becomes my new habit to think about this on my way home. At least for 10 or 15 minutes. So that when I get home, I have a fun challenge. This is not a challenge like at work. This is going to be a fun challenge. Because my new commitment to my body makes it worthwhile. I want to take care of my body."

4

■

Sabotage Due to Expectation of Failure

Okay, _____, take some nice, easy breaths and start to orient to internal experience. Internal terrain for the next while. And just a moment of relaxation is like the word "induction," which means to usher in, as it were. It's like someone opening the door and saying to you, "Here, this is the place where you want to be."

So you put yourself into this different state of mind. Where you . . . feel more comfortable and calm and effortlessly concentrating on what you want to do. Regardless of distractions and alien thoughts that may come. Concentrating on yourself.

You came to see me because you have a problem that we have already defined and specified. And now you want to concentrate on that. Not so much as a problem, but in terms of the solution. How you are going to get out of it?

When you think of yourself in your own personal history, you may remember many times, especially as a child, when you believed in some sort of magic. It was wonderful to believe in Santa Claus. But then, you found out that Santa Claus didn't exist. And you took it from there. Perhaps there were people whom you trusted, whom you thought were perfect. And then they showed their human imperfections.

And there was also one big false belief that you took in, a belief that had to do with perfection. And perfection is one of the biggest lies in the world. Many people still believe that they can be perfect. But the truth is that no living thing can be perfect, because we are always changing. We are always growing. We are always taking in more information. More knowledge.

And at this point, you may realize, intellectually at least, that this is so. That perfection is really a booby trap. But then there is another side of you that keeps saying, "I have to be perfect. And I have to get into these weight-loss efforts and do it perfectly and not fail." And that's okay, because that's part of you too.

However, at this point, you want to give yourself a little time to challenge the idea of perfection and magic that most of us bring from childhood into adulthood. And then, eventually, we have to get rid of this fallacy, or else we are open to a lot of disappointment.

So remind yourself that the beauty of being human is to be

incomplete. We are constantly growing. We are constantly reaching new levels of knowledge. Of understanding. Of health. And check what happens when you think of that. Do you feel any tension somewhere within yourself? Do you have any sort of negative reaction to that? People usually do.

But then go back to that important distinction. The reaction comes from the child in you who doesn't want to give up the false beliefs. The magic. The perfection. The child who may have evidence that there is no Santa Claus, but still wants to believe in Santa Claus.

And say to yourself, "As an adult, I have to accept responsibility for my actions. And I want to accomplish my goals, not by some sort of magic. But by my effort. By my taking one step at a time.

"I'll be happy to see a **general** upward tendency. Even though there are occasional slips and sabotages. And I want to check with my adult self, and let those thoughts slowly sink in so that my child self stops taking over. I don't want to reject my child self, because it's part of me. And I need playfulness and enjoyment in my life. But I cannot let the child run my life. So when I think of sitting up a regimen to get rid of the weight that I don't need, I want to do it knowing that I'm not going to succeed one hundred percent. Knowing that I'm not going to be perfect at doing it.

"And when I use hypnosis to help myself do it, I want to remind myself that **hypnosis** is a **help,** but it's not magic. The child in me still hopes for magic. Regrets that there is no magic. That things can't happen just by some abracadabra magic word, or by snapping my fingers. But the more adult part of me realizes that there is a lot of fun in having the **challenge** to accomplish things in the process.

"Like the artist, who out of a chunk of marble or stone creates a beautiful statue, this is what **I** am doing. I am creating my own body. I am creating my own self. Not through magic, but through patient work. And like the sculptor I have a clear vision in my mind of what I want to accomplish."

Before the sculptor starts to work, there is just a piece of marble or stone for those who don't know what the sculptor wants to create. But the sculptor has a vision. And you want to say to yourself at this point, "I am becoming the sculptor of my own body. My medium is not marble or stone, but my own living flesh."

"And I'm not going to do it by magic. I'm not going to do it without flaw. But I'm going to do my creation. My work. And I will be proud of it. And I have to keep in my mind the **image.** The **vision.** The clear picture of what I want to accomplish. The body I can have. And the body I'm going to have at this stage of my life. Without comparing myself with anybody else. And that vision has to stay in my mind the way it is now, although it may change from one situation to another, from being in formal dress, to wearing ordinary clothes, casual clothes, a bathing suit.

"That vision, very clear in my mind, is going to be like the compass that leads me to where I want to go. So I'll fail once in a while. And I'll take a couple of steps backward. And that's fine, because my general tendency is to continue to go to where I want to go.

"And I can now visit the future. Put myself there a few months from now and look at myself . . . And feel the sense of pride and accomplishment and joy . . . And feel so satisfied when friends, coworkers compliment me, and say, 'God, you look terrific. You lost some weight, didn't you?'

"And I can say to myself, 'I didn't lose anything. I gained. In self-respect. In attaining my goal. So it was good riddance.' The way we feel about garbage. It's the things that we don't need that we haven't really lost. We simply got rid of them, because we had no use for them.

"And there is weight in my body that I don't need. And I really want to get rid of it in order to gain: in health, in self-respect, in pride, in the sense of accomplishment. So much to gain by getting rid of the weight. It's like the sculptor who gets rid of chips of marble and chunks of stone to **gain** the goal that (she/he) wants to accomplish.

"And with this, holding on to that image. The vision of the body that I'm **going** to have. I want to promise myself, once more, that in order to change my false beliefs into a **power thought,** I want to practice this mind exercise again and again.

"The thought that I am trying to digest and incorporate into my life is the thought of **power.** Because perfection, even though it looks wonderful, really diminishes me. It disempowers me. The thought of accepting my humanity, with its limitations and challenges, gives me the **power** to really take control of my life.

"As the sculptor takes control of the piece of marble or stone and **creates** a new reality out of it. Out of my living flesh, I can create the new reality of my body. And I am doing it **now,** because the whole process of creation starts with a **vision** of what is in my mind.

"And so with that, I can relax even more deeply and then slowly let myself return, at my own pace, to the ordinary way of using my mind."

5

■

Saying "No" to Important Others

Okay, _____, take several, calming breaths and let the rhythm of your easy breathing gently rock you into a more comfortable place . . . That's right. And feel that slowing down occurring in your body. Your heart beat. Respiration. Thoughts. Movement. This is a time for you, and you can let yourself value it as you experience its benefits.

Now you want to listen to your own excuses. And yes, what you say is true, there are people around who, with good intentions put pressure on you to eat the wrong things. Remember the slogan a few years back when they tried to convince children to say "No" to drugs? . . . And that applies to many other things.

You may have decided not to eat a particular fatty food. Yet people keep insisting. "Oh, what's wrong! It's just once! It doesn't make a difference!"

You want to remember why you are trying to change your life. And without necessarily getting angry at the people who may try to take you away from your path, you want to use every instance this occurs as an opportunity to strengthen your resolve. To strengthen your desire to do what you decided to do. And there is always fear in change. So it may be scary to take a stand. A firmness against everybody else it seems.

But that's why you're spending a few moments today and every day for the next few months to strengthen your resolve.

And allow yourself to be clear about the reasons you have decided to establish this change in your life. Very gently review the reasons you have. They're your reasons. Other people may not think they're good reasons. But that is only their opinion.

And now that you have reviewed your reasons for establishing this change in your life, get ready for the difficulties. Every time that we want to accomplish something, there are minor or major difficulties, expected or unexpected.

And, of course, one difficulty may be that you're feeling very comfortable and very calm and several of the important people in your life **tempt you.** Insist, "C'mon do it one time. What difference does it make?" You know their words.

If you are not prepared, it's very difficult not to give in to those social pressures. But if you're prepared by rehearsing these situations in your mind ahead of time, you're going to be okay.

So see yourself in that scene. Very clearly create that scenario. In vivid detail. The place where you are. The people who are around you. The type of food that is offered to you, and sort of live ahead of time. Your reaction. Your temptation. Your desire to do it, "Oh, just one time. Just a little piece."

But then think of your resolve. And let your resolve be a strong force that almost transports you to another state of mind when you face this type of temptation. This type of food. Something that is not for you.

A little portion of something else. Yes, filling your plate in a normal way. But knowing that **you** decide what to eat, and how much to eat. And **add to this** that sense of pride and enjoyment. You are doing what **you** want to do. What is good for you.

The function of chefs is to present the most inviting delicacies, so that we are attracted to them as if they were magnets. The function of waiters is to do public relation work for the chefs.

But you appreciate their art. Their skill, without necessarily having to say, "Yes," to everything that is in front of you or is offered to you. And so, get in touch with a new sense of **pride.** Of **success.** Of enjoyment. You have done something wonderful for yourself. And so, you can go to five restaurants or attend five events a week and still keep to your program. **Your** program that you have chosen for yourself.

And think of the example of some of the public officials who have to go to many banquets and attend events almost every day. Recently, in a report on Henry Kissinger, he indicated that he was doing this: He would spend some time before an event relaxing. Looking forward to the event. But **deciding** beforehand what he was going to eat, and how much. And he would be sick if he didn't have a prepared plan, as he was exposed to so much food every day. So, you can use him as a role model, and pattern your behavior according to the example that he and others offer you.

And rehearse this in your mind. Go over it again. The preparation. The thinking. The deciding. And then the actual doing. And this rehearsal will slowly give you an inner strength that you didn't know you had. And with that, you can return to the ordinary way of using your mind.

6

■

Exercising for Weight Loss

Y our breathing can take you to this movie in your mind, where you see yourself doing your choice of exercise. The exercise that you enjoy, and the exercise you can do without hurting yourself, and in moderation. You want to really be there again. Because we can reproduce in our minds any of the experiences we have had in real life.

And you are going to **feel** fully alive. You want to feel that **energy** of your body that is being increased by the exercise. You're going to feel the **freedom** of moving. The pure, carefree joy of the movement. And you're in a pleasant environment. It's safe. It's comfortable. The atmosphere and the temperature appeal to you.

And so while you are exercising, you feel your body coming to life. And, yes, exercising is another way of celebrating life. "And because of this increased awareness of my physical reality, I am **expanding** the awareness of my body and my needs.

"So I'm going to enjoy this in such a way that I start looking forward to the opportunity to exercise. Disciplining myself to exercise at times has a sense of having yet another commitment." But you want to remember that the word "discipline" comes from the word disciple. You want to be a disciple of wisdom. And exercise is an emissary of wisdom.

"So, the exercise keeps me alive. Makes me aware of my being alive. And because of this, I do it, because I enjoy my life. And I want to make my body last. And to make my body last, sometimes, I have to put my body first.

"My body was made to move, and in exercising, I'm giving it the opportunity to act according to its nature. And as I exercise, I feel my body improving. My stamina increasing. It may not happen the first or second time, but slowly I start feeling the changes. Then the consequences of moderate, regular exercise are also seen in the way I sleep. In the way my mind can concentrate. In the way I eat.

"So I want to watch myself, in my mind's eye, exercising. Doing my chosen exercise. Feeling the sweat coming out of my body. And when I feel the sweat on my forehead and my head, that might be my reminder of how exercising is my way of using my head.

"Leading a sedentary life is a way of not using one's head. To respect my body, I have to exercise. To pay homage to my body, I have to exercise. And to **attune** my body to greater health, and greater pleasure, and sensitivity and awareness.

"So my exercise is something that I **want** to do. That I wish I could do more of. And because of this, it becomes a break in my routine and, in a true sense, a minivacation. And what is a vacation, but a way of establishing balance in life? So my exercise can establish balance in my day, in my week. So that everything in my life is in moderation. Just the right amount of work. Just the right amount of play. Just the right amount of exercise.

"And while I'm exercising and feeling all of these changes happening in me, I know that after I finish, I'm going to feel that good, healthy sense of tiredness. But it's not a tiredness of fatigue. It's a tiredness of satiation. Satisfaction. It's a **wonderful** feeling of tiredness after the workout.

"And because I respect my body, I want to give myself some cool-down time, which will **benefit** my body and my mind. It's allowing the process to slowly wind down . . . Then I may want to have some fluid and go back to my routine activities. And I am exercising my right to move in the direction of health. That's the way I want to see it. In that packed sentence. I am exercising my right to move in the direction of health. Physical, mental, and spiritual health.

"And this exercise gives me an opportunity to be more in control. To be more in charge of my life. And this exercise allows me to show my respect for my physical self. For every part inside of me that benefits from the exercise.

"And I want to just stay with that image. That for me, exercise becomes a very positive, constructive, and beneficial activity. And because it's positive, constructive, and beneficial, I'll find the time to do it. So this is the way I want to look at this activity.

"And because I recognize the value of exercise, I want to find the opportunities to exercise. I want to be **greedy** for the opportunities that the day offers me to exercise, because I want to make my body last and I respect the maintenance of my body. And exercise is an aspect of maintaining my body. Keeping my body in tune, in good shape.

"And with that, I can relax further . . . and I can see myself engaging in various types of exercise activities that I may have thought about. Just to get a feel for that particular activity. Enjoying the way my body reacts. And the sweat and the tiredness and the change in my breathing are reminders of my body's reacting positively to the exercise. And that exercise is beneficial, as long as it isn't excessive or forced. It's a way of balancing. Tuning up your body and your mind.

"And I want to become so familiar with these images in my mind that when it is time to act on them, it will be more enjoyable."

And it may be that as soon as you arrive home from work, you feel the urge to become physically active, or maybe it will be the moment you walk out the door at work that you feel this strong desire to exercise.

And just as you are feeling more at ease now, with your breathing more effortless, you know how easy it is to forget what kind of appetizer you had for dinner at a restaurant a week ago, or what dreams you had, or even what some person might have said to you moments before . . . It's that easy to let there be changes even now in what one is aware of and in what one is not . . . That's right.

And people can sometimes forget things they hear even before they hear them, as they find something else in their own current experience of the world to better absorb their attention, such as a dazzling color, or a moment of music in their heads, no less a funny word, or maybe a colorful song that fully absorbs their conscious attention for the next while in a way that allows their unconscious alone to register the important learnings from this trance experience.

And with that, you can gently, easily, return to the common, ordinary way of using your mind.

7

∎

Craving Vegetables/Fruits

Y ou can begin by taking several regular, easy, slow breaths. Remembering how your gentle breathing effortlessly ushers in comfort. And what this new approach to hypnosis does is to try to trigger healthy reactions from the unconscious. And that's what you want to do when it comes to food. So that the signal of hunger that enters your brain is translated differently than before.

It's like someone who has developed bad speech habits. When (she/he) has a thought (she/he) expresses it in poor English. And if (she/he) wants to improve, (she/he) has to learn to translate (her/his) thoughts into acceptable, grammatically correct English.

Up until now, the signals of hunger have been translated into cravings for fatty food. Food that is filling, but not nutritious. Food that creates almost a sense of lethargy. And now you are in the process of learning how to translate signals of hunger into **craving,** not just desire. But **craving** for food that **is** healthy and nutritious. Especially vegetables and fruits.

And many people who got into the habit of eating fatty foods react negatively to fruits and vegetables. You want to recognize that. And it's fine, because we're not simple entities. And when I say, you, I don't mean your whole self. I mean part of you. So part of you has gotten into this craving for fatty foods.

And that's not the smart part of you, because that fatty food slowly undermines the normal healthy functioning of your body. And that less intelligent part of you is the one that has also created some sort of dislike of, or lack of enthusiasm for, vegetables and fruits.

But there is the other side of the "you." The smarter, the more educated. The more responsible part of "you," who knows that too much of the wrong food is damaging, is slow suicide. And that part knows that it's worthwhile to develop the taste for and the enjoyment of nutritious, healthy, natural food. The right food for you. Like vegetables and fruit.

And you might want to think of vegetables, and see what images come into your mind. Perhaps an outdoor market in a small town in some foreign country . . . Mountains of different vegetables with their different colors. Maybe with the sun shining on them . . . Or perhaps, your image is simply a procession of different vegetables that go by your mind.

And feel free to reject the vegetables that you don't like. But acknowledge the fact that some vegetables you do like. And you do like them in different forms. After all, most vegetables can be presented in various ways. I don't know why, but I'm thinking of eggplant or artichoke hearts.

So just allow yourself to watch them . . . And allow the responsible adult in you to recognize that this is alluring, delectable food. This food gives your body the fuel and nutrition that it needs. And you may want to do the same thing with fruit. So again, we have what we call ordinary fruit that we find daily. But then there are more exotic fruits that you can find in a favorite supermarket, or may have consumed in some other country, or in some exotic restaurant.

And let these fruits go through your mind. Imagine them somewhere in the fields . . . Being bathed to a gorgeous luster by a gentle drizzle . . . Being picked. Go with your images . . . And instead of letting that irresponsible part of you reject fruits and vegetables, allow the more responsible part of you to take over for a moment.

And to recognize that this type of food is connected with your health. With tastes and textures that you can look forward to enjoying. So as you realize that you can benefit from fruits and vegetables, you can take advantage of this food. Appreciating that this food grows in the fields and ends up within your reach. Because, yes, there is a connection. In some mysterious way, all beings are connected. In that flow of energy.

We're interdependent beings. And that wiser part of you may gladly recognize that, yes, you can benefit from this new way of thinking about fruits and vegetables. And so appreciate how eating fruits and vegetables could be a way of celebrating life.

And the fatty foods, the foods that bring more fat than nutrition, can be relegated to an insignificant place in your life. "I want to celebrate life. And I want to give my body the stuff of life so that it can continue to be healthy and strong, and feel more energy.

"I want to reestablish a sense of proportion. Up until now, fat has had a much higher priority than it should. Than my body needs. Than my body can use. Now I want to reestablish the proportions, the percentages. And because I **celebrate** life, I want to give my body the stuff of life.

"So that beautiful, ancient toast of 'La Chiam' is not just for when I drink, but can also be used when I do anything that connects me to life. And food can do that. So I want to purify my food. I don't want to ingest food that is a symbol of life, and at the same time, deleterious to my life. The life of my body.

"I want pure food that does good to my body. That gives my body nutrition. Energy. So it's not that I resign myself to eating fruits and vegetables. I'm going to develop a **taste. A craving.** An **enjoyment** of fruits and vegetables. I'm going to allow my creativity to find new ways to enjoy fruits and vegetables. Preparing them in different combinations. I'm going to take in the color of those beautiful fruits and vegetables . . . And the taste . . . Because fruits and vegetables are on this planet for my benefit. I don't want to miss out on them. And so, yes, it's going to be a celebration of life.

"I want to pay attention to the colors of the vegetables. Such a wide range of colors . . . And I want to pay attention to the colors of the fruits. And the different combinations . . .

"And it's fascinating to think that so many great painters have chosen fruits and vegetables for their still-life paintings. There is a beauty. There is a manifestation of life in fruits and vegetables. So I want to imagine myself **assimilating** that. **Integrating** that into my life. So that health, energy, and life become part of me. And that's why you can say 'Yes' to **life.** The fatty foods say 'No' to life. And **slowly,** I'm going to be able to develop the habit of enjoying food that is a celebration of life.

"Therefore, I can imagine now how those proportions change. Before, there was more fat than fruits and vegetables. Now, I see it in my mind's eye slowly changing so the proportion is more **beneficial** to my body.

"And I want to repeat this mind exercise slowly every day. Giving myself free time to do it, until I feel the difference. Until I realize I'm going to be hungry for the right type of food that is good for my body. Instead of having that almost blind attraction to the food that is mostly junk. Mostly damaging to my body."

8

■

Craving: Grains, Beans, Pasta, and Water

Okay, ————, you can take a few easy, relaxing breaths
. . . which is the first step in learning to soothe yourself. It is also
a step in the direction of personal growth. And, since you have
done this before, you may just let your own inner mind bring
you into that wonderful state of mind that we describe as trance.

So food is all around us. We live in a society that has an abun-
dance of food. And at times, we forget how important it is. It's
our fuel. It's our energizer. And what you want to do now is to
spend some time reflecting on food and its connection with you.

You may want to think of yourself eating something that is

healthy and tasty. Perhaps with your family. Perhaps alone. And your mental image brings you into a place that is very relaxed. Very comfortable. Everyone is in a peaceful mood.

You may imagine yourself talking to your family. Perhaps you are discussing food. How well it tastes. Where it was bought. Where it was grown. Discussing your appreciation of low-fat, nutritious food.

"And a handful of rice in my plate is a link to history. It may come from faraway places. It may have involved an **army** of people to make this handful of rice possible on my plate, and then in me. The people who planted it. The people who collected it. The people who cleaned it, and so on.

"So, in a sense, through food I am **affirming** my connection with humanity. I think that every time I stir a cup of soup, in a sense, I'm stirring the effort of labor and good intentions of perhaps hundreds of people who gathered and cleaned its ingredients. So I want to think of eating food as a wonderful experience. A meaningful experience. We don't eat like animals. Animals just eat to fill their bellies and to get fuel. But we associate most important events with a shared meal. And so many religious holidays and occasions are centered around a meal.

"Many celebrations—anniversaries, birthdays, weddings, bar mitzvahs—involve an important meal. Because the food is symbolic of life and our connection with the rest of the world. With the people around us."

So in that image of eating a meal, alone or with your family, you hear yourself talking about this theme. None of this is really new, but it's good to remind ourselves. And you begin to view food with a different attitude. An attitude of respect. You start welcoming food, not just as a material thing that makes the life of your body possible, but as a spiritual thing that has a meaning. That has symbolism.

And you start to crave the type of food that is friendlier to your body. Low in fat, or without fat. That is easier to digest. And you start **craving** food that is more directly connected with nature: grains, rice, pasta, beans. The more processed and cooked and worked on the food is, the more we forget that it's basically coming from nature.

And you can enjoy **more** . . . a lesser amount of food, because you're enjoying not just its taste and its nutrient value, you're enjoying its meaning. Its symbolism. And with this, the idea of water comes to mind. By drinking water, we affirm our nature. Most of the planet is water. And so you may wonder why we call it "Planet Earth." And by drinking water, it's as if I'm affirming, once more, my need to be a part of the planet. So I let water cleanse me. In many religious rites, water is a **cleansing** symbol. As a way of purifying, not just the body, but the mind, the soul, the spirit. So water will be, to me, purification. Pure means without complicated detours. So that I can have a clear, direct vision of my being. My essence as a human being.

"And so my body will celebrate life by eating pasta, grains, rice, beans. And by taking this **inner** symbolic purification by **increasing** the amount of water I drink. Because the water puts me in connection with the real world in which I live while it purifies me, and helps my body function at its most effective level.

"And the final thought that I want to keep and I want to share with every cell in my body is that I want to celebrate life by doing the ordinary things, like eating more natural foods and drinking water, and in a more meaningful way.

"I have this wonderful privilege that other beings on this planet don't have. Of thinking. Of discovering and appreciating the meaning of symbols. And I want to use this ability when I eat. When I drink more water. So that I feel **the** joy of being more alive. So that I feel the joy of making my body last. Because this is the only body I have. And the means that allows me to be alive. To be in touch with this wonderful world in which we live.

"And this attitude will **ooze** out of me toward the people with whom I'm in touch: friends, relatives, clients. So that my celebration of life will enrich them, and will help them not to miss out on this tremendous opportunity that we have. In the meantime, every cell in my body is receiving this message of joy, celebration, meaning, because I'm alive. And with this, I may want to spend a moment or so just relaxing a little more and letting myself go to an even more comfortable state of mind, looking forward to my next meal. To my next opportunity to really celebrate my being alive."

9

■

Slowing Down the Act of Eating

Let the relaxation slowly enter into your body, as your breathing slows down all of your bodily functions. Your heart beat. Your breathing itself. And with that, imagine yourself eating alone. But not in a hurry. Not standing up. Not distracted. Just eating.

The time has come. You're alone and you want to watch yourself in your mind's eye sitting down. You have set the table. And you have taken out the food and, instead of **attacking** the food as so many people do, take a moment to become aware of it's presence (presents). Become aware of the miracle that's going to take place in a few moments when these portions of food that are on the plate will become part of you. Part of your very tissues and blood and flesh.

So with that attitude, you realize that eating can be a very meaningful experience. There is an element of intimacy. Of closeness. Of communion. So after that moment of concentration, feeling that the food is your friend, because it's doing something good for you. It's keeping you alive and in good health. The food that you have chosen because of its healthy qualities.

After that moment of concentration, you then start this wonderful experience of eating. In some Eastern countries, they conduct an entire ceremony around the simple pleasure of drinking a cup of tea. You want to imagine yourself going through some sort of ceremony or ritual around the very basic need for food. Not that you're going to do this every time you eat, but you want to do this once in a while to remind yourself that you can really slow down the eating experience.

One of the problems many people in our culture have is that they eat too fast, too much, and too frequently. If you capture the beauty and excitement of eating, almost as a ritual, then you will realize that you won't fall into that trap of eating too fast, too much, and too frequently. Many religions make meals a central aspect of their beliefs and rituals. You want to make your meal a central aspect of your living. Not that you live in order to eat. The opposite is true.

So you want to see yourself there. Lifting the silverware you use to eat. Almost caressing the food while you are getting some of it to put into your mouth. Admiring the different textures, aromas, shapes, and colors of the various foods, and allowing that food to become a part of you.

And as the food enters your mouth, you become aware again of the texture, the shape, the temperature, and then how that temperature changes as it is warmed by your own body temperature. And as you chew it, how the texture changes. And then as you swallow it.

And that, in a sense, is where the mystery begins, because all that you have done so far has been done consciously: the selecting of the food, the putting it into your mouth, and the chewing. But when you swallow, you are involved in an act of faith, trusting your inner mind to take care of this food. And in a few hours, this food, which on the plate was something definite, becomes part of you. Of your flesh, your body, blood, tissues.

The process, of course, starts when you look at the food, smell the food, appreciate the food, place it in your mouth. When your saliva flows to wet the food to make it digestible. And then when you swallow the food, you're going to become more aware of those sensations, just to be more in touch with the **mystery.** To recapture a sense of **awe** and admiration.

And to achieve what you want, you allow yourself time. Knowing it's better to eat less in a slow way than to gulp a lot of food just because you seem to be in a hurry. So you **slow** down. And because you slow down and become more aware of this wonderful mystery that has taken place and has taken place since you were a baby, you want to **respect** the process.

So the food that's in your mouth has to be chewed, has to be tasted, has to become part of you. You befriended that food.

45

Then you swallow it. And **only** after swallowing that first morsel, do you put another morsel of food in your mouth. Again, you may have observed people in public places. How they fill their mouths. How they don't chew enough. How they are distracted from the process of eating.

You want to concentrate on the process of eating. Because you want to **rediscover** a new value, a new lesson, a new opportunity to grow, to be in touch with the mystery in life. And so you don't want distractions. You don't want to eat and read a paper or balance your checkbook, or listen to the radio, unless it is soft music that complements your eating.

And also since you are alone in that image, that movie that you're watching, you are not talking. At times, people get involved in heavy discussions or idle chatter while they're eating. And, again, that distracts them from the process of feeding.

And an interesting thing to remember is it seems that we are the only beings on the face of this planet that have the privilege of becoming aware of the importance of the eating process. Other living beings just eat. But we can give meaning to this very simple, primitive activity.

And still watching yourself enjoying that food more than ever before, because you're slowing down. You're looking closer at a beautiful, complex picture. You are acquiring a new respect for this process. And because of this, every part of your body, in a sense, is involved. Your breathing is altered while you eat. Your blood pressure changes. The level of sugar in the blood changes.

Many muscles in the body are activated, and others relaxed.

And you realize that this is an opportunity you have a couple of times a day to really be fully aware of your being. The food is a friend, an associate, a partner for living. Without food, you can't live.

And, consequently, you want to treat this food as a friend that you respect. As someone you are paying attention to. Someone you are greeting with real joy and enthusiasm. And you want to stay with this thought that, yes, your meal can be a celebration of life.

And then when you're familiar with this picture of yourself eating alone, you may add other people to the picture: family, friends, associates. And again, even though you are paying attention to them, it's like background music, because your main focus is on what's happening between you and the food. This food that is presented on the plate is not yet a part of you. But it will become a part of you in a few moments.

And so even though you are with other people whom you enjoy being with, that other theme is playing in the background. Not as a distraction, but as an enrichment. And what better opportunity to enjoy being alive than when we are with people we care about and who are a part of our lives.

So food is a partner of living. And so, I remind myself, "Food is a friend who allows me to go through this journey of living. And the whole process of feeding myself is a real mystery. And the food that I eat becomes my very being. In a sense, once the food is digested by me, it changes its name. Because it becomes me.

"And reviewing the way that I can ideally eat, the way I can eat once in a while, I see that to do it in this more ceremonious, more ritualistic way can slowly change my attitude so that I never allow myself to **gulp** food down. To eat indiscriminately. To eat without thinking, without reflection.

"And then the reality will change, because my attitude has changed. And the reality will be that I will feel **sated** more quickly than before. I will enjoy the food more. I will discover more tastes. More nuances of taste, enjoyment. And that will make me feel more alive.

"And if I change my attitude toward eating, eating slowly, I'll change my attitude toward other important areas of my life, because eating is one of the most primitive activities, one that we cannot avoid. So if my attitude is more respectful, that will expand to other areas of my life.

"With this, then, I want to go back to my breathing. Allowing myself to relax. Another primitive activity, breathing, that I can make enriching and meaningful. So that the breath of life gives me the opportunity to grow as a person. To become more aware of who I am. Yes, the breath leads to breadth.

"And while I'm still relaxing, I may want to promise myself to go back to this tape and practice this again so that I can truly get to the point where I have a different attitude toward food. Where I am going to benefit my health and my spirit in general because of it. And with that promise to myself, I can interrupt this activity knowing that I will return to it as some other point."

10

■

Food for Self-Definition

Okay, _____, take the effortless, easy, deep breaths that have helped you to reach levels of relaxation that you really have come to appreciate. And you can reconnect to one of the pleasurable sensations that you experienced here in trance . . . And you can be curious about what other interesting sensations you will experience in this trance.

And then spend some time thinking of food . . . "Because food is my friend. My savior in a way, because food keeps me alive. But I recognize that I have given food a more powerful role in my life than it actually should have.

"I don't want to use food to fill a type of loneliness or empti-ness. Food has a physical function in my body. I use food for my benefit. My body knows what to do. I just put the food in my mouth and then my inner mind takes over, without my having to be concerned about what happens next.

"But at times, I let food extend its power, and instead of being limited to my physical well-being, it oversteps its limits and gets into the area of my emotional well-being. And I want to correct this right now. I do not want food to fill an emotional void inside. Because that is not the nature of food. And it's a very easy escape.

"I want to be honest with myself and recognize that emotional emptiness and loneliness have to be filled in an emotional way. And for the time being, that's all I need to remind myself of. That emotional emptiness requires an emotional filling. I'm not going to create this strange short circuit, where something like food that serves a very important and powerful function in my life is used for something else.

"It makes as much sense as a drunk enjoying his wine so much that he decides to pour some of it into the gas tank of his car, because then the car is going to enjoy it too. I don't want to fill my emotional void with food. So I cannot allow food to define me. Food is my servant. Yes, I called it a savior. But it's like a servant-savior. Food works for me. For my benefit, and I cannot allow it to take over.

"The food in my belly does not decide whether I am alive or real or not. I want to go to my true emotional sense and work on developing that further, rather than to confuse the issue and create more problems by accepting food as my self-definition.

"So I want to see myself, in my mind's eye, eating a good meal. Enjoying it and eating with an attitude that is positive and optimistic. I'm not eating to satisfy some emotional need. I want to think, while I'm seeing myself eating like this, of the healthy ways of satisfying my emotional needs. In my relationships . . . In my work . . . In my attitude toward the world . . . In my sense of humor.

"And all of these things are not directly connected to food. So I want to work on myself in all those areas that have to do with my emotional well-being and **cutoff,** once and for all, this confusion where I'm using food to define me rather than to nourish me.

"Yes it's true we are one, and my soul is a part of my body and my mind is not limited to my brain, but that doesn't mean that I have to create confusion. My body is a good metaphor for the order of life. There is a special place for each organ. There are special fluids and functions in each part of the body. And some of those fluids that are very beneficial in one part of the body can be damaging if they enter another part of the body.

"So the same is true of my whole life. The food that is very beneficial to my physical health and well-being can become very dangerous if I allow it to enter the area of my emotional well-being. Yes, I can look at my body and use its functioning as a metaphor, or the order and hierarchy of functions. And I can then transfer that order to my life as a whole. It's true that I am a unit, but it's also true that I have my physical self, my intellectual self, my social self, my spiritual self.

"And I want to be sure that these things don't get confused, as I have been doing by allowing food to become a means of satisfying emotional needs. The order of things keeps everything moving. And I see this not just in my body, but in any type of machinery. In every social system. In every hierarchical system.

"And I will make things easier for myself by respecting that order. The old Romans used to say that if a person respects the order, the order will protect that person. If I respect the structure of things, the structure of things will benefit me. And that applies not just to my material being, but to my whole being.

"I'd like to jump ahead in time and imagine how wonderful it would be to enjoy food for its own value. For its nutritional effects on my body. While at the same time, I have a satisfying time in my relationships. In my work. In my social life. In my sense of self-esteem and self-respect.

"I want to step into the future. Experience myself in that way, because this is the way I can be. This is the way I want to be. And this is the way I shall be. But only after I establish this order in my life. And I can stay with that image of myself. And I can stay with that enjoyment of life that I can have and I will have in the near future. And in order to make sure that this will happen soon, I can promise myself to practice this mind exercise again and again, until I have established that food is my friend for my physical needs and that I want to keep it there within that order. And with the promise to myself to practice this again and again, I can then slowly bring myself back to the ordinary way of using my thinking powers."

11

■

Lacking Resolve:
When Eating Away from Home

Okay, _____, take some nice, easy breaths . . . And let your breathing lead the way to a relaxed place and space in which you can gently place yourself. And you are already in a place that you have selected to take better care of your body. To be slimmer. To get rid of the weight that you don't need and are carrying, like someone carrying a heavy suitcase.

And you have found that there are certain situations that make it difficult for you to stick to your resolve. And somehow cause you to **revert** to the old eating habits. You know those situations. It may be a holiday. It may be a dinner with some friends. It may be eating in a restaurant.

And so, what you want to do is to use this mind exercise as a vaccine to immunize yourself against that particular danger. What do we do when we are given a vaccine? We train our bodies to react with antibodies against a disease. So you now want to train your mind. Your body. Your spirit. Your whole self to create some mental antibodies. And in order to do this, you have to prepare yourself. Like the vaccine is a preparation to ward off the possibility that the disease may come.

And the preparation is simply for **you** to plan. For **you** to decide. And the decision is not based on some sense of obligation. Rather, it's the sense of pride. If you are the only American in a group of foreigners who may not be very friendly toward the United States, you may have a sense of pride in being an unofficial ambassador of the United States.

So that is the way you behave. The things you say. The tolerance you show, helps them to realize that perhaps their idea of what America is, or what Americans are all about, can be changed.

So you want to prepare yourself to realize that even though you're surrounded by temptation, **you** are in charge. You can decide how to handle the situation.

But before you are tempted by temptation, by a holiday or a celebration, you can prepare yourself. It's interesting to see how many people plan so carefully when it comes to doing things that are unimportant to them. But when it comes to food, they don't plan. They just let themselves drift helplessly into the situation, and then they are **tempted** and do things that later they will regret.

So imagine yourself, not necessarily at the event where there is plenty of food, but preparing yourself. Thinking about it. Giving yourself a few minutes to say, "Yes, I know what I want to eat. I know that at a family gathering, instead of having five pieces of some rich food that I like, I can have one or none.

"At a restaurant, if the person I'm with has some rich food that I like, I can ask if I can have one piece. And I can eat it slowly and savor the taste. And I can pick other delicacies, according to my taste."

Then go to the situation in your mind's eye, go to the restaurant. And at times, it may feel that the food surrounds you. That you're in the middle of all this delicious food.

But you know that you want to have a good time **now** and tomorrow, when you think about it. And you have prepared yourself. And you have decided what you want to eat. So watch yourself going through the choices on the menu, saying, "No to this. No, I'm not interested." Taking one portion of this. A little portion of something else. Yes, filling your plate in a normal way. But knowing that **you** decide what to eat, and how much to eat. And **add to this** that sense of pride and enjoyment. You are doing what **you** want to do. What is good for you.

The function of chefs is to present the most inviting type of delicacies, so that we are attracted to them as if they were magnets. The function of waiters is to do public relation work for the chefs.

But you appreciate their art, their skill, without necessarily having to say, "Yes," to everything that is in front of you, or offered to you. And so, get in touch with a new sense of **pride.** Of **success.** Of enjoyment. You have done something wonderful for yourself. You can go to five restaurants or five events a week and still keep to your program. **Your** program that you have chosen for yourself.

And think of the example of some of the public officials who go to many banquets and other events almost every day. Recently, in a report on Henry Kissinger, he indicated that he was doing this: He would spend some time before an event relaxing. Looking forward to the event. But **deciding** beforehand what he was going to eat, and how much. And he would be sick, or dead if he didn't have a prepared plan, as he was exposed to so much food every day. So, you can use him as a role model, and pattern your behavior according to the example that he and others offer you.

And rehearse this in your mind. Go over it again. The preparation. The thinking. The deciding. And then the actual doing. And this rehearsal will slowly give you an inner strength that you didn't know you had. And with that, you can return to the ordinary way of using your mind.

12

∎

Being Overweight to Punish Oneself

O kay, _____, you can start giving yourself the pleasure of very comforting, self-soothing, deep breaths . . . Easy and regular breaths that you can feel occuring very naturally . . . So that soon, it feels like your body is breathing you.

And you can say to yourself, "I want to be in touch with my weight. With my physical self. With the image I am projecting with my physical self when I am in front of other people. And I want to remember, that yes, this is me. And this is my body. And I want to accept my body, even though it is not yet the body I plan to make it.

"So like entering a home when it's very messy and dirty, I don't reject the home. I improve the home. And I start slowly, one corner at a time. To make it organized and clean. So my being in touch with myself reminds me also of my responsibility. I want to be proud and have a sense of being kind to myself. Responsible to myself.

"And since I realize that my weight has colors and tones of self-punishment, I want to focus on that more clearly right now. Because once I find this key false belief, this myth about myself, I can go to work and sculpt the body that I not only want, but the body that is my birthright.

"It's like the doctor who finds a tumor that may be malignant. He doesn't let it spread. He attacks it. Extracts it. And frees the body from this tumor. My false belief, that I need to be over-weight to punish myself is going to be the focus of my attention. Because since it's a **false** belief, I want to get rid of it. And in a sense, I don't want to spend too much time figuring out how it started and who contributed to this false belief becoming a part of me. I want to get rid of it. But I want to convince myself that this **is** a **false** belief.

"In primitive times, people thought that thunder or earth-quakes or other natural phenomena were indications of God's anger. And they offered sacrifices and they did ritual dances. Then with the advance of science, humans realized that those occurences were natural phenomena. They had to do with the laws of nature of our planet.

"So they realized that all the sacrifices and dances and rituals were completely disconnected—had nothing to do with the natural phenomena. So now in my life, I have been acting as those primitive people. Using my excessive weight as a way of not being the way I can be. Of punishing myself.

"And that false belief, that I don't deserve to be at a more comfortable weight, that a more comfortable weight is not meant for me, is what I am now **dispelling.** And I want to get in touch with myself. I've been **cheating** myself for years because of this false belief.

"So this false belief has been like a **traitor.** Like a **saboteur** . . . in my life. And **now** that I have **unmasked** it, I cannot just look at it and say, 'Oh yeah, that's part of me. I want to get rid of it. Like a country gets rid of a **spy** who has been selling important secrets to another country. They don't say, 'Oh, those things happen.' They get rid of it.

"So the punishment is going in the wrong direction. I'm punishing myself and I'm punishing everyone I know, because everyone I know is **affected** by my extra weight in some way or another. When the punishment should go **against** this false belief that has **crept** into my life and has become part of me.

"I need radical surgery on my mind, in a sense. And I can imagine myself doing that. That false belief is lodged somewhere in my brain. I can perhaps visualize it in some part of my brain. And that false belief can look like some strange-looking animal or insect that has roots and connections. So I can do a little bit of mind surgery and go to that false belief and extract it. Cutting off all its roots, so I feel the **relief** of having gotten **rid** of that false belief.

"And I can pay close attention to that **growth** inside of my mind. Obviously, we're not talking about a physical, but a mental, reality, like a metaphor. And that's why I want to focus on this more and more. Because I want finally to free myself of this false belief that has made me a **slave.**

"I have accepted the control of my weight over my mind. And I want now to get **rid** of that belief. And with it, slowly free myself to get rid of the weight I don't need. And **if** that belief has lasted for many years, it doesn't mean that I have to take a long time to change it. Once the spy has been uncovered, (she/he) is kicked out of the country or executed.

"Once I recognize my false belief, that I need to punish myself with my excessive weight, I say, 'This is absurd.' I have done unnecessary harm to myself. And if I want to undo mistakes of the past, I can undo them with good deeds, good words instead of punishing myself—in a sense, bad deeds against myself.

"And I want to send that message to my inner mind, I **do** deserve to be thinner. I **want** to do this for myself to make up for the many years I've used that false belief **as** if it were true. And as a result, I've stagnated in that brackish pond of excessive weight. So now I want to see myself moving. Once that growth of that false belief is removed from my mind, I can imagine all the other positive thoughts flowing without that obstruction, because that extra weight has become a drag. Has slowed me down. And I am stuck. So I want to move. And let's get in touch with all the images of movement. Of progression. Of advancing. And let my mind be filled with those images . . . Of graceful movement. Of smooth movement. Leaving behind the ugly images of that false belief that had **stopped** me. Talk about dead weight. Yes, that was the weight of death. Now I want to get rid of it and have the freedom of growth and life.

"And I want to feel good about it. And in order to do so, I want to put myself in the future for a few moments. Rehearsing the way my life will be when I am not acting under the influence of the false belief. I am free . . . And if I have to make up for past mistakes, I'll find good ways of doing it. And I'm going to protect myself so that I will **never** use myself for punishment.

"Yes, I can make up for past mistakes, by doing good for people around me. By offering my talents, my services, my gifts. But I'm not going to **desecrate** my body by using **it** for punishment. And I can go back to those primitive people who were sacrificing to those angry gods based on all their false beliefs. And often there were human sacrifices. And this is what I've been doing. Engaging in this human sacrifice. And now, I'm **stopping** it. As those human sacrifices were stopped when knowledge and understanding of the laws of nature helped people realize that those primitive beliefs were absurd. So I want to be in the future and **see** myself in my mind's eye first, so I can then do it in reality. **Acting without** the false beliefs. **Accepting** my body the way it can be at a much more comfortable weight. And enjoying life without being **stuck,** staying in that overweight condition as a way of punishing myself. I'm free at last, and I can move on now. And in order to **undo** the wasted years of my past, I want to practice this."

13

■

Compulsive Eating as a Defense Against Feelings

Okay, _____, take some nice, easy breaths . . . And look forward to another experience of enrichment and personal growth. And, ultimately, trying to gain greater mastery. Greater power. Control. Over your life. And yes, you have a problem with eating in a compulsive way.

Instead of just having one little spoonful of ice cream. Savoring it. And finding all the sensuality in the taste and texture of it, you have to have a whole pint. But the truth is you don't have to binge. You can learn to enjoy food without using it to escape something. To build a wall between you and something else.

And you may want to ask yourself, "What is that something else? What am I trying to separate myself from? Or what am I trying to bury, to cover up?" Ask yourself that question. And use the image of separating yourself from something else by means of the food . . .

Then use the other image of covering up. Burying something . . . And even now, your inner mind may be bringing some notions. Some ideas. Yes, we can use food to keep ourselves alive. To renew our energy. To be in contact with the world. But we can also abuse food. Without the balance of moderation we can use everything against ourselves. Water, for instance, is absolutely necessary for existence. But you can drown if you are in too much water.

"So I would like to open my mind now. It's like I want to have a disciple's attitude. A student's attitude. I want to learn. But the interesting thing here is that I am learning from myself. My inner mind. In other words, my conscious mind is opening up as a student. As a novice. And the teacher is my own inner wisdom. The wisdom that I've accumulated through the years. Even before my birth, since we know that the fetus is already picking up messages and learning before the actual birth.

"And I can take a quick look at my lifeline. All these years. Every day I've learned something about myself. About life. About the world. But the things that I learn as a human being are not just facts put into a computer. Every fact comes wrapped in some feeling. Some subjective reaction. Some emotion.

"However, as I often do with gifts I've received, I unwrap the gift and I throw away the paper. Instead of admiring the paper.

Recognizing that it has a beauty of its own. That it must have been chosen with great care and deliberation to enhance the gift itself.

"I have done the same with many of the things I have learned. Thrown away my feelings, my emotions. From the facts. From the events. Throwing away those emotions. Disregarding them. Ignoring them. And trying to stay with the facts.

"But in so doing, I have cheated myself. In ignoring my feelings, I have shortchanged myself. And I want to use this opportunity to recognize, first, that, yes, my feelings exist. And second, to recognize that my feelings are important and deserve my attention, because they will enrich me. They will fulfill me. They add meaning, color and dimension to what otherwise is a black-and-white, flat picture of living. And last, to recognize that what I've done for a long time doesn't have to continue for the rest of my life. From now on, I can make up for lost time and really be in touch with my feelings. Knowing that feelings are friends, and you don't abandon your friends.

"So what I want to do is allow my inner mind to continue sending the messages that it sends with my feelings. But from now on, I want to pay a little more attention to my feelings. Recognizing that my feelings are part of me. I want finally to grow up and stop having the attitude of the boy who says, "Oh, these feelings are for little girls." Feelings are **sexless,** in the the sense that they belong to humans. Not just to men or women.

"And to be the most fulfilled human being I can be, I want to welcome my feelings and pay attention to them. It doesn't mean that I have to be constantly concerned about my feelings, but to pay attention to them.

"For instance, when I feel that need to eat something I know is not the right type of food and I know it's not because I am really hungry—when I feel that need, I want to get into the habit of waiting. And checking. Almost in an expecting way. Not to analyze. Not to figure it out. Just waiting. Again, like the student. Like the novice. Like the disciple. Is my inner mind trying to tell me something? And what is it trying to tell me?

"I have bad habits, just as every human being has. And one of them is that the moment I think of food, I have to have food. But now, the moment I think of food, I want to wait. I want to give myself a little time to check to see if the message that my unconscious is giving me comes to me in a different way.

"I have gotten into this habit of using food to separate myself from something, or to **bury** something. Now, I want to slowly change that. And it's like learning a new skill. Much like every new skill we learn, in the beginning, it's a little difficult. It can be uninteresting. But I want to think of the end result. I'll have more control of myself. I'll be more aware of myself. I'll have more inner-power, and then I can make more choices. Otherwise, I'll be like an iceberg for the rest of my life. Just aware of the surface above the water, without realizing there's a tremendous energy buried inside the water belonging to the same entity.

"So my program is very simple, but now I want to convince myself that I can do it. And I want to imagine myself the next time that I am tempted to get the type of food that I don't need.

I want to visualize myself in that situation. And instead of going like an automaton, like a robot, to the place where the food is stored, simply because I **thought** of the food, I see myself saying to myself, 'Wait a moment. I can wait. I want to stay with myself. I want to connect with my breathing. I want to do a little bit of what I'm doing right now.'

"And perhaps I'll better understand what this is all about. If there is no physical need for the food, if there is no physical need for the amount of food, it is a **bad** habit that I've gotten into.

"And rather than understanding its origins and tracing its history, I simply want to get in touch with it so that I can get past this habit to the real reason for it. The real cause of it. Which **may be** some feeling that I am avoiding or minimizing. Some feeling that I'm afraid of, that makes me uncomfortable.

"And by rehearsing this mentally, I'm making it easier for me to handle it when it happens again, maybe tonight. Maybe tomorrow. So **I** want to **extend** my control, my power over my life. And then **if** I decide to have that food that I don't need, it will be just a little snack. Just to satisfy my taste. To enjoy it to the fullest. Without having to **stuff** myself with it.

"And it's interesting to think what will happen if I take one little nut, for instance, instead of a handful, like most people do when they eat peanuts. Just one. And taste. And savor. And extract all the sensuous and tasteful aspects of it.

"And I want to do it just because it enriches me. Giving me more color, a new dimension. A new sense of meaning that I have never enjoyed before. And yes, I want to watch myself in my mind's eye, in great detail. Being **able** to stop myself. And to say, 'Hey, it can wait. I don't have to rush to get the food just because I think about the food.'

"One memory. One idea. One thought gets me going. Why not change that thought? And I want to change that thought and say, 'It can wait. I can relax. I can take a couple of nice relaxed breaths.' And check what happens. What is this yearning for food covering up, if anything? What exists behind this blind, desperate yearning for food. I'm getting curious. I want to know. **Then** I can do something about that it. But I don't want to react automatically by **separating** myself from that feeling, or by **burying** it, **covering** it up.

"So in the next moments, I can let these thoughts sink into my whole being. I can imagine these thoughts echoing in my body. In every cell. After all, every cell is affected by the food I eat. So I can imagine, in a cartoonlike fashion perhaps, that every cell becomes like a sound box that is reflecting these thoughts. Every cell joining in this effort to **break** that habit. To change that habit. And to enjoy that moment of relaxation . . . waiting. Expectation between the thought of food that I don't need, and the action of going to get it. And I can visualize the cells in my brain saying '**Yes**' to this idea, and the cells in my heart, and all the millions and millions of tiny cells in every part of my body all the way to my fingertips and toes and earlobes. '**Yes**'. And I want to have that '**Yes**' attitude. Yes to new possibilities Yes to life. Yes to this curiosity that has started in my brain right now. Finding out what's behind that. Asking myself why should I miss out on something that might be interesting, enriching, meaningful.

'Yes,' and with that yes attitude every time I say to myself, 'Yes,' I can imagine that message that I have been giving myself going deeper into my very being. Touching every organ. Getting into every organ—my heart and my liver and my kidneys and my spleen and my pancreas.

"Yes to this new attitude, which is really a cry of freedom. I want to be free of my old habit. I want to liberate myself and declare my independence from this habit that has sneaked into my life with my barely realizing it. And then all of a sudden, I feel trapped. But I want to change that feeling. I am not trapped. I am now learning the way to become free. 'Yes' to that freedom. And with that, I can now allow myself to return to the ordinary way of thinking."

14

■

Overeating in Response to Denial
of the Body's Changing Needs

Okay, _____, you can take several nice, deep breaths and begin to feel yourself shifting your focus to a more internal place that you can gently move into. A place that feels safe, secure, with endless possibilities of interest to you. And letting your breathing be your guide down to that special place.

Much is being said about keeping our bodies young, and misconceptions abound. Imagine your body right now . . . Imagine yourself examining your body . . . Look at the way your body is, from toes to head . . . And notice of course, that even though this is the body you had as a baby, a child, an adolescent, that body has changed.

The body is not like a machine that just wears out. The body is constantly regenerating itself, rejuvenating itself. So give yourself a chance to examine every tiny detail of your body. You can start with the surface of the body . . . And now imagine some sort of fantasy trip inside your heart, your liver, your kidneys, your spleen, your pancreas, your digestive system, your lungs, your brain, your bloodstream . . .

You want to get to the point where you realize that your body is serving you well. Is constantly working to keep you alive. **But** this is not the body that you were given when you were born. This is not the body that you had when you were 10. This is not the body that you had when you were 15 or 25.

The body changes. So you don't want to think of it as wearing down like a machine. This is a living entity, and it's too bad that we only focus on our chronological age. The body has a biological age that is related to the health of its systems.

That's why we may see an adolescent who is unable to function well. Whose biological body is much older than his years. And at the same time, we see someone in her 50s or 60s, whose body **is** biologically younger than that of other people at that age.

So what you want to do is have a new respect for the fact that your body is in a constant process of change. And that to want to force your body to be the way it was in the past is insulting, injurious to the body. You don't want to act now as though you are 15 or 25.

There are changes that we go through in each stage of our life that present us with many pulses and many minuses. Especially if you look at the whole picture of the body, the mind, and the spirit.

So let your inner wisdom pick it up from here. Let your inner wisdom recognize what's going on here. "I'm fooling myself if I think that at my age I can do things as I did when I was 10, 20 years younger. I have to **respect** the changes in my body.

"In a sense, yes, this is the same body I had many years ago but it's also completely different, because all my cells have been changed. Cells grow and complete their function and new cells are created that reproduce themselves. So I want to respect the changes in my body. Not with a sense of regret, but with a sense of curiosity, adventure. Now I have other opportunities that I didn't have before: physical, mental, and spiritual opportunities. I have new social opportunities, in terms of relating to other people, using my experience, my wisdom. And in order to be fully alive, I don't have to stay as I was 10 or 20 years ago. In order to be fully alive, I have to be fully in touch with the reality of myself now." At times, we see those **fools** who at age of 50 still want to act like their grandchildren aged 15. "I don't want to fall into that pathetic way of looking at life. I want to recognize that the changes in my body are new opportunities to experience new things that I was not able to experience as a child or as an adolescent or as a young adult.

"Aging should be saging. Not thinking, 'I'm losing ground,' but feeling more grounded. The idea of being rejuvenated doesn't mean that I want to be as young as I once was. I want to have the attitude of openness to life. Of excitement over new opportunities, and the curiosity about the unknown that I had as an adolescent thinking about being an adult.

"And that old song about love's being 'a many-splendored thing,' applies to life as well. It applies to me, to my many experiences in life. To my many stages in life. Each stage has unique pluses and unique minuses. **But** I want to train my mind to focus on the pluses, and **accept** the minuses. The things that I had when I was much younger are not things that I have lost. Instead, I have traded them for new things that I can use now that I was unable to use when I was younger. Wisdom is one thing that comes to mind. So life is largely a series of trade-offs.

"So I want to **enjoy** who I am. Being my age, and being fully healthy and involved in life at **my** age. I don't want to act a child's age. I want to accept who I am and I want to enjoy being who I am. And as I said before, I want to trust my inner mind. To let my inner mind bring me to my reality. Bring me to my senses. I don't want to waste any more energy lamenting what was left behind. Regretting that I can't be as physically energetic as I was in the past. But look at the things that I have now. The opportunities that I have now. The wisdom. Experience. Respect from others.

"And with this new acceptance of myself, I can also accept the fact that my body cannot get rid of the fat I put into it the way it could when I was (a young adult/an adolescent). And that's why I have to eat low-fat foods. Foods like grains, vegetables, fruits, and beans. In other words, I find myself wanting foods that are low in fat and high in nutrition.

"Being _____ (current age) has many pluses, but I can no longer trick myself into believing that one of them is being able to get rid of the fat I put into my body as I could when I was (a young adult/adolescent).

"At _____ (current age), my overall bodily needs have drastically changed from when I was _____. So now, knowing that I have to do more to get rid of weight, and striving to sage as I age, I can remember not to forget to remember to be more protective and disciplined in my eating patterns.

"And with this, I want to look **forward** to the future. Keeping myself in good shape is my responsibility. Doing the things in my life that are reasonable in terms of food, exercise, rest, and balance. And my goal is to remember that my body now has different requirements than it had when I could take off the weight more easily.

"And in order to change my attitude, I can promise myself that, yes, I want to practice with this tape regularly. So that I can **accept** with joy and pride and gratitude who and what I am today and what my body needs today. And with that, I can bring myself back, slowly, to the ordinary way of using my mind."

15

∎

Using Food as a False Symbol of Family Unification

Okay, _____, take some time out to bring yourself into the slowing, gentle, soothing rhythm of relaxation. And let your breathing become your tour guide into the state of ever-developing calm.

And you can now begin to remember some of the myths that some families have that to sense the unity in the family, food is necessary. I guess the concept of the religious idea of communion relates to that. At least today, the whole concept of communion has to do with food.

And what I want to do now is to really **challenge** that myth.

Food has to do with survival. Period. But we can add all sorts of meanings and symbols to food. And so for some people, food has to do with communion with the divinity, with some sort of god up in the sky. And the way to get close to that god is eating that particular food that has been specially blessed for that purpose.

In some other religions, people had sexual communion with specially blessed people or animals representing the divinity. Whether it is through sex or through food, the whole thing is absurd, because food is not a vehicle for communion with any divinity.

But I am doing the same thing if I accept food as a symbol of acceptance and belonging and unification within a family. Actually, I didn't invent this idea, it came from my family, and maybe my parents accepted it from their parents, and it may go back through many generations

So the reality is that by using food in this way, I may be stopping myself from the real feelings that may exist within the family, and within myself.

And then, paradoxically, the food that is supposed to unite us becomes a barrier to the real feelings. We're so involved in eating and sharing the meal that we become less sensitive to each other. Less caring about each other. Less concerned about each other's inner life.

So if food has nothing to do with love and acceptance, food has the meaning that people ascribe to it. Some people kill with food, by poisoning the food. Therefore, it's as ridiculous to say the food is a sign of hatred as to say that food is a sign of love.

Food is a physical necessity and in that sense, yes, it's a friend of mine because it keeps me alive. But I can then add the superstructures of love or hatred or divinity or communion or family unity. But what I want to do is trim food from all this symbolism, and just view it in its beautiful essence: an energizer that's keeping me alive, strong and fit. The rest, is superimposed.

And the family unity has to do with attitude, help, mutuality, concern. The family may be very close and united, even if they never share a meal together. And, yes, I know that once I have a clear idea of what food does for me in my life, I can **enjoy** a meal together with friends or family. And then the atmosphere of that meal becomes one of unity and contact and acceptance and love. But it's not because of the food. It's because of the attitude.

So I want to recognize that by holding onto this false idea that I received as a child, I'm acting like the people who believe that food can be a bridge or union with some divine Being. This is as **erroneous** a belief as the one that **most** people in our society recognize as crazy—that some sort of sexual activity can be a means of union with some sort of divinity. So I can imagine myself getting rid of that belief. Extracting it from my mind, or kicking it out of my life. And feeling free to enjoy food for what it is. Not with some **deceptive attitude.**

And feeling free to take advantage of the benefits of food, without these superimposed meanings that people since time immemorial have been ascribing to food. Food is food and I want to take it for all its value, but without the other vacuous connotations. And I want to unblock myself from all these other myths that create so many complications. I want to be at peace with myself and I want to be content with myself and to enjoy food at its best for my benefit.

Yes, my family may have conveyed some distorted ideas about food, but now as an adult **I** can look at them again and recognize, yes, that was a mistake. And their way of looking at food very often **blurs** feelings, and blurs closeness and union. And by **freeing** myself from all the faulty connotations connected to food, I can really begin to more fully enjoy being part of my family, and more connected to my feelings.

And I want to repeat this practice again and again, because I'm trying to change something that has been instilled in me since I was a baby. And it takes a little bit of effort and perseverance and repetition to **really** change this old, outdated maladaptive attitude.

So with that desire to repeat this practice again and again, I can now bring myself back to the ordinary way of using my mind.

16

■

Weight-Loss Determination for the Impulsive and the Passive Client

Okay, _____, take a few of those easy, deep breaths. And let your mind and your body remember that feeling of comfort from your prior trance experience here . . . how it felt to feel freer. Being able to let go more than you may have thought you would. And the other sensations you associate with comfort. Maybe it was a growing warmth . . . or a soft coolness. A lightness . . . or a heaviness . . .

And ask yourself why you want to get rid of the extra weight. Why you want to have a trimmer body. And wait for the answer that comes from you . . . What I am suggesting is that the answer has to be your own conviction. Not to please others. Not to feel safe in the old body image that you have had and people know. But **your** own personal reasons and decision.

And you have thought about it. You have read about it. Ultimately, it has to do with feeling better. Making your body last by protecting it from the foods you know are not beneficial to the body.

So you want to think of yourself as healthier, because you want to help your body last. Because you want to avoid possible malfunctionings of the body, which we call illness or disease. You want to be **actively** involved in your **effort** to attain your goal. To have the body that is best for you. In terms of health. In terms of energy. And, yes, in terms of appearance.

You want to be actively involved in protecting your body from the bad habit of eating foods that may satisfy the passing urge, but fail to benefit the body in its very complex functioning. And to be an active participant means that you **know** what you are doing. So think about it now. Imagine yourself, for example, learning to understand a little more about nutritional labels. Imagine yourself in a store reading these labels and understanding them. Knowing what they are saying. Because they are affecting your life. Thanks to this knowledge that you are acquiring, the quality of your life can be improved.

So you want to remind yourself that you want to become more knowledgeable about nutritional information, because the food that the labels refer to is going to affect your body. One way or another. Once you put some food into your mouth and swallow it, it affects your body.

After all, your body is like a helpless, little baby. Once **you** decide to feed it something, it processes it through the same mechanism with which it would process any food, good or bad. You could actually take poison and the body would start processing that poison as if it were food, and you die.

So visualize yourself reading a nutritional label. And this makes you feel more in charge. And **then** the by-product of this is that you are going to have a more sophisticated attitude. You see some food. Very attractive in its packaging. With colors. With shapes that are attractive. And then you read those nutritional labels and you find out that the food is **junk.**

So you might become **angry** at the food **manufacturers' deceptions**. They are trying to lure you into submitting to their intentions, which are to make money. **Disregarding** your **health.** Disregarding your well-being. So you become angry as you would at anyone trying to deceive you into parting with something you cherish.

So you want to imagine yourself, again, right there in the aisles. Where you buy the food. Recognizing that many of these products are very elegantly packaged. Very beautiful to the eye. And the contents may not be good for you. And you watch yourself, in your mind's eye, taking one of these packages and reading the nutritional label. And becoming **angry.** Becoming **furious** at these food manufacturers for insulting your intelligence by trying to seduce and deceive you. Creating a situation that is a trap into which it is very easy to fall.

They present food as if it were friendly and beneficial for you because of its attractive packaging, but in reality it is an enemy that, if allowed to, will infiltrate your body to do damage in the short or long term.

So let this attitude be yours. You enter the store as an area that is almost like a minefield. Full of traps. And you're going to use your intelligence. Your knowledge. To check those labels. And not to be deceived. Your weapon against deception is your intelligence. And you want to be there with that **weapon** ready to be used. Because you have the right to protect yourself.

You want to assume full responsibility for your body's health. And you're not going to let the manufacturers of food use you in their quest to make money at the **expense** of your well-being and your pride. So, in a sense, you go into the supermarket as you would go to a sleazy area of the city. Where dangers may be lurking at every doorway. At every corner. You are there with **great** alertness, awareness. Taking precautions. Prepared.

The food aisles are full of danger, because they can **activate** your old impulsive desire for fatty food. The old habit of buying things.

So think about yourself. It's almost as if the child in you who grew up developed these bad habits of buying food that looks good without knowing or appreciating enough its nutritional value. Now as an educated adult who uses (her/his) intelligence to protect (herself/himself), you want to protect that child. You're not going to let that child run through the aisles of the store, just as you wouldn't let a child run freely through a dangerous area of the city. You don't want to be the victim of crime. So to avoid being the victim of crime, you have to take precautions. You have to avoid certain areas completely.

And your **weapon** is your knowledge. No one can take that away from you. You want to use that knowledge and you want to become more educated and more aware of food content. You want to be an educated consumer. You want to be a sophisticated consumer.

Think about this question: Why do you resist getting rid of the extra weight? If you're truthful with yourself, you may discover that there are some fears. It's a risk. Your appearance will change. The reactions of others will change. So it may seem easier to stay in a position that's familiar and seems safe. However, you want to summon your inner conviction and say, "I can handle the changes. I can be more attractive. I can be thinner. And yes, people will notice me more, but I know how to handle it. With a smile. With a nod. As a validation of what I have accomplished out of determination and conviction. And as a result, I'm gaining a new sense of pride. A new sense of control over my own destiny. And my most important tool is my intelligence, and my determination. And at this moment, I want to make a pledge to myself, that I am not going to be deceived by food manufacturers. They don't know me as an individual, but they know that many people are ignorant and impulsive, and react to the way the food is presented, to the slogans. I won't let myself succumb to the seduction. So my pledge is that, from now on, "I'm not going to put anything into my body unless I know what benefits it will give me. I need to know the food is a friend before I invite it into my body. So my task now is to **challenge** those ways I had of deciding what to eat.

"My pledge is, 'I want to learn more about nutrition, and to consistently read nutritional labels, so that I don't put any food into my **mouth unless** I first know how it will affect my body.' And that will give me a sense of freedom. Of being in charge. Of being **above** all this brainwashing that takes place as a result of misleading food advertising.

"And before I finish, I want to remind myself that this is a quantum change in my attitude. Consequently, I have to reprogram my mind by repeating this tape again and again. Until **I** recognize that my attitude has changed. And that my sense of self-protection doesn't allow me to eat any food without first knowing what it really consists of. Its ingredients and nutritional value.

"And that will make my eating more joyous. Because **I** am deciding what I want to eat. It's like choosing my friends, or choosing where I'll go on vacation. I want to have that attitude toward my food. I am going to decide what food to eat. Not just because it's on the shelf. Not because I saw some advertisement on TV, but because I know this food is good for me. So I am really **my** own boss. I became the master of my own life. My own destiny.

"And with that **sense** of freedom and exhilaration, I can slowly bring myself back to the ordinary way of using my mind."

17

■

Compulsive Eating as a Defense Against Anxiety and Depression

*Before the induction, get three to five power thoughts from the client. A power thought is defined as a self-empowering, positive statement concerning one of the person's goals in his or her hypnotherapy work.

Okay, _____, take a few, easy, deep breaths, which is a preliminary to . . . becoming relaxed. We start with the idea of, yes, you take care of your body. You know when you need some way of changing the way you're feeling. You may be overly anxious. So you want to do something about it.

You may be overly depressed and you want to do something about it. What this mind exercise does is train you to do the healthiest, most helpful thing for your anxiety, depression, or any other state of mind, as we call it. Actually, it's a state of feeling that you are experiencing.

So, just before you start, become aware of your physical presence. Of your body. Allow that sense of protection. Of love. Of caring to increase in you. Every little part of you is important. Every nerve. Every cell. Every organ is important, because it's part of the whole.

At times, I think of this when I go over one of those big bridges. That every little screw and bar has a function, and that it would be very dangerous for the safety of the whole bridge to just say, "Oh, I can take this off and I can change this."

So allow that sense of **respect** for your body to become very clear in your mind. And at the same time, to realize all of the complicated functions that are taking place in your body this very moment and every moment in your life, from conception to the end of your life. Allow that sense of **awe** to come to you. "**I** am a living **miracle.** I'm a living **marvel.** Every walking person is a **mysterious** event." And with that, go back to yourself. And say to yourself, "Yes, I not only have the right to do something about some uncomfortable feelings that I may have. I have an obligation. My conscious mind must be responsible for my well-being. But the thing that I have to remember is to learn **which** is the healthiest remedy for my distressed feelings.

"And I realize I have used the wrong type of remedy, as I use food not to fuel my body so that every part of my body can function at its best, but very often I use food to hide my anxiety, my nervousness, my fears, my depression. And that's not the right function of food.

"If my car needs gas, I'm not going to pour perfume into it. If I am anxious or depressed, food is not the right remedy for it. Even though, on the surface, it make me feel okay, the only reason it makes me feel okay is that it distracts me from the real issue.

"So I want to learn to apply the healthiest remedy to that special condition. And the healthiest remedy is not from the outside. Not from food. But from the inside. From my own thoughts. I want to develop **power** thoughts that will **enable** me to **cope** with the anxiety and the depression better.

"I will enlist those power thoughts that very often will be powerful enough to lessen the anxiety. To change it. To allow me to go back to a more comfortable and content way of being."

And which are the power thoughts? Before today's trance, we discussed the idea of having some sort of journal of thoughts that are powerful for you. And after you write a list of five, ten, or more of these power thoughts, you can let them come to your mind when you start feeling anxious or depressed. So let's use the power thought you came up with here today, which was, "The solution to my anxiety or depression comes from me. I have the remedy from **within** to resolve my anxiety. I don't need outside influences to resolve my anxiety." And just let that power thought sink in. Another power thought might be, "I have the resources in me to cope with this anxiety. I don't need to rush to get some food or other distraction."

And many people who are called **addicts** are people who got used to an unhealthy way of coping with their anxiety and depression. And the problem is: It doesn't work. And that's why they need more and more of it. And the situation never improves.

So you want to **develop** these power thoughts. "**My** anxiety is controlled from within." That's a power thought. "I have the power in my mind to control my anxiety, my depression. I **can** control my anxiety and depression, **without** reaching out for food. And once that thought has become part of me, it becomes much easier to handle the real situation."

So you want to rehearse this in your mind. You want to imagine yourself in a situation where you are anxious or depressed about something. And you just came from food shopping and have a refrigerator full of food. But **imagine** yourself doing the helpful thing. The healthy thing. Because your power thought becomes reality. Your power thought is translated **into** action.

And what your **power** thought says is, "**All** that wonderful food has nothing to do with my anxiety. The **remedy** for my anxiety is in my own mind." And in this movie that you are watching that shows what can happen. This movie of what **will** eventually happen. You see yourself doing other things than medicating yourself with food. You see yourself taking a couple of nice, comfortable, deep breaths. You see yourself organizing your thinking. So that you do what is in your power to do in terms of this situation that creates the anxiety/depression. You calm yourself down, so that you take a little distance from this situation that seems to be **impinging** on you. And you give yourself some **true,** positive statements about yourself. "I have experience. I can handle it. This is going to be difficult. I don't like it. But I know how to do it. I can plan. I can organize my thinking."

And instead **of letting the anxiety/depression take over, you** control it. It's like a plane that is caught in the middle of a storm. Instead of staying at that height, it usually moves higher. Moves away from the storm itself. And you can imagine yourself like that plane, looking down on the storm from a higher altitude. What a spectacle. How beautiful. But it doesn't affect the plane because the plane has moved away from that storm.

You can imagine yourself removing yourself from that anxiety storm . . . And instead of reaching out with the old, ineffective habits of the past, reaching out for food, you move away from the anxious situation by taking control of your body. Of your breathing. Of your relaxation. And engaging your mind in effective ways of thinking about the situation that creates the anxiety/depression.

And the more you think about it, the easier it will be to accomplish it. This is mental rehearsal. A skater who wants to perform in public has to rehearse for many hours. You want to do the same in your mind. Rehearse **the new, effective,** cleaner way of resolving your anxiety.

And let the movie continue. At times, you want to put it in slow motion. So that you see yourself in every little detail . . . doing the helpful thing. And **not allowing** yourself to reach out for food to resolve something that food is not meant to resolve. And allow the movie to come to an end. A **satisfactory** end. Where you feel **great** about having done it in the helpful way.

Where you feel **proud** of yourself. You feel accomplished. And you can truly say to yourself, "This is terrific. I've done something that I'm very pleased with. Happy with. Proud of . . ."

And with that, just relaxing even deeper for the next while to collect all **your energy, your determination.** And now **oriented** to the things you want to do after this practice. So promise yourself to use this tape faithfully. Every day, because you want to be **free** of the old habit of reaching for the **wrong** remedy. And start using the old remedy that works, which is in your thoughts. In your mind. In your imagination. And with that, you can then go back to the ordinary way of using your mind.

18

∎

Weight-Loss Plateaus

Okay, _____ spend a few moments with some of those easy, deep, regular breaths that you are becoming accustomed to. And let that more relaxed breathing gently usher in that state of inner strength and control.

And imagine yourself on this plateau, and what comes to mind? It may remind you of those mesas in New Mexico. Those huge, flat mountains. Very few people have been there, but once you're there, it's like an unending parking lot. Or you may have the image of sailing. You're away from shore and there is no wind whatsoever. But the day is gorgeous. Because usually when there is no wind, the day is nice. What other image comes to mind? Those are the two that come to my mind.

The first thing is to fully accept that I find myself on this plateau. And I need to get in touch with my feelings. What's happening here? Am I giving myself some negative self-hypnosis. Am I saying there's something wrong with me, I should be moving forward? Am I impatient? Am I saying to myself, "I don't have time for plateaus," I have to move forward.

So you can be aware of any negative self-talk. And you can substitute it with telling yourself that plateaus are part of nature. The whole universe as far as we know has cycles, and some of the cycles are very active. Others are very passive.

A plateau is part of the cycle that is passive. So there is no plateau if there is no process. The only time we avoid reaching a plateau is when we are dead. So just the idea of being on a plateau is a very positive one. "I have done something. I have started a process. I have gone to some point and then it levels out for a time."

So you can realize that the plateau is not a final result, but a step in the process. It's like someone who is jogging. There is one split second when the body is not touching the ground. It's air-bound. Well, nothing to be frightened about, because this is part of the process. If we could see it in slow motion, we would realize that the person is in the air.

So part of you will say, "I'm disappointed. I don't like this." But you want to appeal to the realistic, intelligent part of you that says, "If there is no plateau, there is no process. If there is no down, there is no up.

"So I have to stay with that faith **in the process and in** myself as part of the process. And I have to **quiet** the childish and unrealistic and impatient voice that is overreacting to the plateau. In a true sense, I should welcome the plateau, because it's a reminder of my being in the process and my doing something positive within the process.

"And that's why I want to prepare myself for the next plateau, so that I can welcome it. I can recognize that this is what being human is all about. I can recognize that the plateau not only is inevitable, but is enjoyable. It puts me into an acute awareness that this particular weight-loss effort is the correct thing for me to do.

"If I were always in the active or up stage, I would have to wonder what was happening. It would be like winter all year round. It's not natural. And my preparing myself for the plateau is going to be a celebration of this growth. I don't want to focus on the plateau itself, because, by itself, the plateau doesn't make sense. But it makes sense within the context of the process.

"So when I start feeling uncomfortable with the plateau, I want to take a few steps back and look at it as if from above.

"Someone may look at a parade at the same level as the people marching and here the person is looking at one or perhaps two people in the parade. But if one could watch the parade from the top floor of a high building, one would be looking at the parade as a whole or as one.

"And I want to look at my life and my progress from the top of that building. Realizing that sometimes there are spaces in the parade. It seems as if the parade is finished, but no, another group comes along. If I'm just standing on the same level looking at the parade, I may be confused and say, 'Oh, it's finished.' But if I am looking from the top of the building, I realize there may be even a whole block of nothing, but that the next group is not far behind.

"So I want to work on my own images that have to do with this process. With this progress. And it's like in music, the silences in the music are as important as the music itself. Otherwise, there is no distinction.

"And with this, I can let my inner mind associate freely and go back to my initial image of being on the plateau. Where am I? What am I doing? What are my feelings? If I'm still feeling impatient or disappointed, I can go to my more rational self and let that part remind me, 'There's nothing for me to worry about.' And then I can relax again and bring myself back to the ordinary way of using my mind."

19

■

Weight Loss: Feeling Deprived After a Successful Effort

Okay, _____, you can take several easy, relaxed breaths and begin to orient toward the idea of self-growth, self-improvement, enjoyment. Allowing the breathing to become very natural . . . Very spontaneous.

And with that, you want to review what you have been doing for your benefit to maintain your body in good health. There are certain machines in our technological society that require constant maintenance, but the effort is worthwhile, because they save us so much time and produce a vast array of valuable benefits for us.

And what you're doing with your body is similar to that. And I think it would be helpful for you to spend a moment just giving yourself some credit. Recognizing that you have put a lot of effort into sustaining healthier eating patterns. And try to think of it as something very positive. You're doing something for your health. For your looks. For your sense of pride. For your sense of being in charge of your life. And feel good about it. Congratulate yourself for having sustained this low-fat eating.

And maybe you can imagine some sort of a trip through the main inner organs that benefit from this effort. You may start with your brain. And there are so many complex structures and organs and systems and glands in the brain . . . Perhaps going along the spine, now . . . Going through different organs in your chest: your lungs, your heart. But take your time, because the important thing is for you to recognize that this **effort** is worthwhile . . . And you can imagine that you are visiting all these parts of you to hear their reaction.

You have favored every part of your body by maintaining the low-fat eating. So you can be delighted and you're feeling proud, recognizing that your inner organs have appreciated this effort. That they give you credit for it. Because, in a sense, every part of your body is like a helpless, little baby. If you don't take care of it consciously, it can be damaged.

So you have been the guardian. You have been the protector. And every part of your body is thanking you. And once you finish this trip inside your body, you can then feel a new sense of **fulfillment**. You have **done** something you set out to do. You had a goal and you followed a process to accomplish it. And that, in itself, is your main focus of attention.

Yes, at times, you have felt deprived. Yes, at times, you yearned to be able to do whatever you instinctively wanted to do. **But** that's not the whole of you. And it may be very helpful for you to remember that. That you can focus on that part of you that has done something **positive.** That has done something important for your own benefit.

Let those thoughts sink in . . . And then remember that even though you are an adult, there is still a rebellious, childish self with whom you will have to contend forever, like everyone else does. And perhaps you want to focus on that right now. Appreciating that it's as if there were two people in you. The one who says, "If I see the fatty food that I like, I'm going to have it and the hell with everything else. After all, I've sacrificed enough. I suffered with this." And so on.

And then, the other part, the part who says, "I am entitled. Not to the food that harms me, but to my **success.** I am entitled to **finish** what I have begun. And I am not going to allow that immature, rebellious part of me to distract me from my challenge. I am not going to let the immature, rebellious part of me undo the work that I worked so hard to accomplish."

Again, visualize the immature/rebellious part of the self. Visualize yourself very sharply in your mind's eye. The way you look. Your size. Your hair. The way you're dressed. Your jewelry, if any.

And remember, you are this part also. So this is you. You want to take care of this part, but in the right way. The way an adult takes care of a child. Very often, **that adult may have to deny** the child some of the things (she/he) wants to do. To **forbid** (her/him) to do certain things. Because the adult has a **wider view** of the consequences. Of the future.

So be sure that you can visualize yourself in that aspect of your personality. The rebellious, immature self that says, "I want it, and because I want it, I have to have it." And then in the same picture, let your mature you step in . . .

You are not going to have an argument. You are simply going to **persuade** the adolescent. **Convince the adolescent** you to cooperate. And let the adult, more mature you have that sense of certainty that says, "Yes, I can handle this kid. I can take care of this kid. I love this kid, because (she/he) is a part of me. And I know that (she/he) gives me a hard time and wants to take over my power, my control, my authority."

So imagine yourself having this conversation, where you are **convincing** the childish, immature self of the compelling reasons to **move away** from that temptation when the craving for fatty food **seems** irresistible. And there is a very simple mental trick to make the irresistible come under your control. The trick is to just **not** focus on it. **Not** to think of it as the only reality at this moment.

And think about this **strong** body that you want to have. About the **healthy** body that you want to have. Think about the **health forces** in **you** that are unimpeded by the absence of excess fat. And, yes, you have made a sustained effort, but that's an **added** reason to say, "I am not going to let anything **rob** me. **Burglarize** me of this goal."

So the one who sabotages your efforts is you. But not your whole self. It's the immature, rebellious self. Perhaps your rebellious (child/adolescent) self. And when you start feeling that **craving,** that desire to have food that you know is not good for you, address yourself to the (child/adolescent) self.

And make an effort **literally** to turn your back. Go to another room. Go to the bathroom and stay there for a couple of minutes, remembering the (child/adolescent) in you. Looking at yourself in the mirror and seeing not just the adult self, but that rebellious, immature, young (girl/boy) who is trying to take over your control.

And with a smile and a sense of love and protection, you can remind that part of you, "I won't let you destroy yourself. I won't let you destroy your goal. And I do this because I love you. And I do this because I want you to be proud and healthy, and disciplined. Otherwise, you'll be like a yoyo. One day feeling proud and on course. Then, when temptation comes, going back and sabotaging. Then later, feeling dejected, depressed. You want steadiness, consistency, because you can get to like that inner peace. That pride."

And you may want to consider the possibility that some little voice inside you is making you feel guilty for almost reaching your goal. Having done something **good** for yourself. And that voice may have come from the past. From messages that you got from, perhaps, well-meaning people, or not so well-meaning people.

"So that those messages I have been giving myself will be transmitted to every part of my body. And especially to that part of my brain that may still be under the control of my immature, rebellious self. Causing that program in that part of my brain that has to do with desire for food to change. And every time I practice this mind exercise . . . that program is changing.

"So that then I can be surrounded by **mountains** of the fatty food that I'm tempted to have. The most attractive, delicious, well-prepared food that I want to have and I **know** is not good for me. And I can feel **proud** by saying, 'The hell with it. This is not for me.' And **walk away.** I want to visualize that scene, rich with color and dimension. Because I know that very soon, this is going to happen for me.

"These thoughts are taking over, so that my whole body is **geared** in that direction. My body **prepares** itself to act according to the thoughts that I put into my mind. And these thoughts will translate themselves into action. These thoughts **will** become my reality.

"And, yes, I will have my (child/adolescent) part, to have fun. To enjoy life. To be adventurous. But **never** again to **damage** myself."

And with that, slowly and at your own pace, you can bring yourself back to the ordinary way of using your mind.

20

■

Being Overweight as an Expression of Passivity/Hostility

As you are moving into this special mind activity, you are giving yourself a present. And stop for a moment to think about that, because a little voice inside of you may say, "Oh, I don't deserve a present. I shouldn't give myself a present. But the present you give yourself is in accordance with the whole mystery of being alive."

If you believe in God, there is a reason, from God's point of view, why you are alive on this part of the planet at this moment. If you don't believe in God, you still look at the mystery of life. The seasons. The order in the universe. And you are part of it.

You cannot isolate yourself, because you need the air that is part of this atmosphere and you need the temperature and you need the correct atmospheric pressure.

And you are influenced by things that come from the earth and become part of your life through food. And the whole planet is in balance, because of the influence of the position of other planets of our solar system in the galaxy. So think about this moment as a little break in your routine, where you **connect** with the reality and the mystery of your life.

And the reality of your life is that you are unhappy with your weight. That you know you are overweight. That you say to yourself that you **should** get rid of the weight.

That you have some fantasy or hope or expectation that makes you believe that once you get rid of that extra weight, your life can be better. Your life can improve. **But** somehow, you stay with that extra weight.

So you may want to recognize that beside the part of you that says, "I need to lose weight," there is another you that holds on to that weight.

The you that has become so familiar with that weight that it now believes that this is part of your being. So it's as if you are now splitting yourself into two different sides of you, like a coin has two sides. On the one side, you're saying, "Yes, I must lose weight." But, on the other side, another part of you is saying, "No, this is me. I can't lose weight. I won't recognize who I am if I lose weight."

So what you want to do during this mind exercise is to change that false belief. Your weight has nothing to do with your identity. This false belief is as harmful as someone saying that because she grows older, she's losing her identity. Your identity is more fundamental, more important than your weight.

So **challenge** your false belief, and notice how that false belief leads you to engage in **ineffective** decisions, which are decisions to eat the wrong foods, to eat too much food, not to exercise. When you deceive yourself into believing that you're hungry and deceive yourself into having a snack.

So this mind exercise will help you to change your false belief. And the first step is to recognize that this is a false belief. The second is to start challenging it. And the third is to let that false belief go, and with it, all the ineffective decisions associated with it. All the ineffective decisions you make that are associated with it. Let the more intelligent part of you look at the situation and say, "I get involved in routines, habits, that require the lesser of two efforts.

"And I have to put my foot down and say to myself, 'I'm not going to eat just because I think that I am hungry.' From the point where I'm at to starving is a long, long way. So I don't have to think that I will starve; that's another false belief. I'm going to check my language too, so that I don't psyche myself into believing, 'Yeah, I'm starving. I can't hold on for another minute.' We know that the body has a lot of resources, especially when we are overweight. There is a lot of fat that the body can use to sustain itself for perhaps several days.

"So **my** attitude, 'I can help it. I have to be fat,' is one of the attitudes that I really have to challenge and change. My intelligent part may recognize that this attitude has given me an excuse not to live my life more fully. This attitude has given me an excuse not to take risks, such as meeting people socially and professionally. 'Oh, I'm too fat. I can't go to this party. Oh, people are going to look at me.'

"So I want to listen more to my intelligent part that has suspected for a long time that those are false beliefs. And I want to get rid of my false beliefs. I want to **discover** my real body underneath all this extra weight and fat. Because I want to do this, I'm going to become the guardian, the protector of my own health. And the guardian of my own health is going to remind me, 'No, you're not starving. You're not dying for a piece of candy.'

"And I'm going to call my own bluff, recognizing that very often I act like a spoiled, little brat who can't wait and can't say 'No,' and wants what she wants when she wants it. I need to start using some of the principles of tough love with myself.

"And tough love means **real** love, without spoiling. Without giving in to whims and wishes and caprices.

"And I want to be tough with myself in order to live more effectively. More productively. In order to be healthy. In order to enjoy longevity in good health. It's about time that I **shed** all this extra weight that is slowing me down.

"That I use as an excuse not to participate more fully in the adventure of living. And, of course, while I think of this, I know that I have to tune up several other areas of my life. The way I eat. The way I exercise. My attitude toward myself. This is what I'm working on now, my attitude toward myself. I have to convince myself, and the first step is to repeat it to myself, 'I am worthwhile. I am important. I deserve respect from myself and others.'

"My body is not a garbage can where I throw in all sorts of junk food. My body is a living mystery that has to be handled with care, like a very delicate piece of machinery. I want to get to the point, **today,** while working on this tape, where I stop fooling myself. To be honest with myself. To say to myself, 'If you want to do it, do it. If you don't do it, stop saying to yourself that you want to do it, and recognize that you are lying to yourself.'

"Yes, I am being a little harsh on myself, but I want to honor that part of me that is intelligent. That knows what's going on. I don't want to continue any longer through life acting as if I were completely fooled by the false beliefs that I use against myself. In a sense, what I am doing now, even though it sounds tough, is to take my side. To take the side of life. I don't want to go on through life fooling myself, underexercising, overeating.

"I am separating myself from my old destructive eating habits. Separating myself from all these unexamined, false beliefs that I've been taking in as if they were true. So in a true sense, the enemy has been myself. That side of me that has acted as if this were my destiny, that I'm going to be fat for the rest of my life. And I can't help it.

"My **destiny, that I declare** today, is to be healthy. To enjoy life. To participate in the activities of life. It's up to me, and that's why I have to keep an attitude of watchfulness. And that's why this tape will help me. So I want to listen to this tape every day, until I realize that I am changing my attitude. And with this change in attitude will come other changes in behavior. The way I eat. The way I exercise. The ways I have used my body that have not been kind to my body, like overeating and underexercising.

"Up until now, I have let myself drift aimlessly. From now on, I am taking over. I am controlling my destiny. So, in order for this to become a reality, I want to practice with this tape every day until I notice a change in my attitude. Until I notice a change in my behavior. And with this, I can bring myself back to the ordinary way of using my mind. Knowing that tomorrow I'll be practicing by doing this mind exercise."